# Handbook of
# Pediatric Neurology
# and Neurosurgery

# Handbook of Pediatric Neurology and Neurosurgery

**Sarah J. Gaskill, M.D.**

Division of Neurosurgery, Department of Surgery, Duke University Medical Center, Durham, North Carolina

**Arthur E. Marlin, M.D.**

Clinical Professor, Department of Pediatrics, University of Texas Health Science Center at San Antonio; Chief, Division of Pediatric Neurosurgery, Santa Rosa Children's Hospital, San Antonio

**Little, Brown and Company**
**Boston/New York/Toronto/London**

**Library of Congress Cataloging-in-Publication Data**

Gaskill, Sarah J.
   Handbook of pediatric neurology and neurosurgery/Sarah J.
Gaskill, Arthur E. Marlin.
      p.      cm.
   Includes index.
   ISBN 0–316–54639–9
   1. Pediatric neurology — Handbooks, manuals, etc. 2. Nervous
      system — Surgery — Handbooks, manuals, etc. 3. Children — Surgery —
      Handbooks, manuals, etc. I. Marlin, Arthur E. II. Title.
   [DNLM: 1. Nervous System Diseases — in infancy & childhood —
handbooks. 2. Nervous System Diseases — surgery — handbooks.   WS 39
G248h  1993]
RJ486.G35  1993
618.92'8—dc20
DNLM/DLC                                                          93–19182
for Library of Congress                                               CIP

Printed in the United States of America

EB-NC

Sponsoring Editor: Nancy Chorpenning
Production Editor: Kellie Cardone
Copyeditor: Joanne Hebert
Indexer: Julia Figures
Production Supervisor/Designer: Madeline Belliveau
Cover Designer: Jennifer Niederst

# Contents

# Preface

Clinical pediatric neuroscience is unique. The neurological problems of children are quite distinct from those of adults in their management, treatment, and outcome. *Handbook of Pediatric Neurology and Neurosurgery* was conceived to guide and instruct medical care givers in the recognition and management of pediatric neurological disease.

The basics of pediatric neurology and neurosurgery are covered in a manner that is useful to a wide audience, including pediatricians, pediatric neurologists, pediatric neurosurgeons, neurosurgeons, neurologists, family physicians, and students. It is not intended to be a definitive text, and surgical technique is not discussed. Rather, it covers the basics of clinical pediatric neuroscience from the developing embryo through childhood and adolescence. Emphasis is on the *recognition* of disease patterns and their appropriate *management*.

We hope that this handbook will serve as a useful reference for physicians who treat children.

S.J.G.
A.E.M.

# Abbreviations

| | |
|---|---|
| AA | Amino acid |
| ABC | Airway, breathing, circulation |
| AChRP | Acetylcholine receptor protein |
| ACM | Arnold-Chiari malformation |
| ACTH | Adrenocorticotropic hormone |
| AFP | Alpha-fetoprotein |
| ALL | Acute lymphoblastic leukemia |
| ASD | Atrial septal defect |
| ATP | Adenosine triphosphate |
| AVM | Arteriovenous malformation |
| AZT | Zidovudine |
| BAER | Brainstem auditory evoked potentials |
| BEAM | Brain electrical activity mapping |
| +/-C | with and without contrast |
| CEA | Carcinoembryonic antigen |
| CIDP | Chronic immune demyelinating polyneuropathy |
| CIE | Counterimmune electrophoresis |
| CMD | Congenital muscular dystrophy |
| CMV | Cytomegalovirus |
| CN | Cranial nerve |
| CNF | Central neurofibromatosis |
| CNS | Central nervous system |
| CP | Cerebral palsy |
| CPK | Creatine phosphokinase |
| CSF | Cerebrospinal fluid |
| CT | Computed tomography |
| CVA | Cerebrovascular accident |
| DMD | Duchenne muscular dystrophy |
| DTR | Deep tendon reflex |
| EDAS | Encephaloduroarteriosynangiosis |
| EEG | Electroencephalography |
| EMG | Electromyography |
| EMS | Emergency Medical Service |
| ENG | Electronystagmography |
| ESR | Erythrocyte sedimentation rate |
| EVD | External ventricular drainage |
| FDG | Fluoro-2-deoxyglucose |
| FSH | Follicle-stimulating hormone |
| FSHMD | Facioscapulohumeral muscular dystrophy |
| FTA-ABS | Fluorescence treponemal antibody absorbtion |
| +/-G | with and without gadolinium |
| GABA | Gamma-aminobutyric acid |
| GBS | Guillain-Barré syndrome |
| GFAP | Glial fibrillary acidic protein |
| GH | Growth hormone |
| HC | Huntington's chorea |
| ß-HCG | Beta-human chorionic gonadotropin |
| HIE | Hypoxic-ischemic encephalopathy |
| HMSN | Hereditary motor and sensory neuropathy |
| HSAN | Hereditary sensory and autonomic neuropathy |
| HSP | Hereditary spastic paraplegia |

| | |
|---|---|
| ICP | Intracranial pressure |
| IM | Intramuscular |
| IQ | Intelligence quotient |
| IV | Intravenous |
| IVH | Intraventricular hemorrhage |
| LH | Luteinizing hormone |
| LP | Lumbar puncture |
| MEP | Motor evoked potentials |
| MG | Myasthenia gravis |
| MLF | Medial longitudinal fasciculus |
| MRI | Magnetic resonance imaging |
| MS | Multiple sclerosis |
| MSUD | Maple syrup urine disorder |
| MVA | Motor vehicle accident |
| NADH | Reduced nicotinamide-adenine dinucleotide |
| NCV | Nerve conduction velocity |
| NE | Norepinephrine |
| NF | Neurofibromatosis |
| NG | Nasogastric tube |
| NMEP | Neurogenic motor evoked potentials |
| NTD | Neural tube defect |
| OPCA | Olivopontocerebellar atrophies |
| PDA | Patent ductus arteriosus |
| PET | Positron emission tomography |
| PKU | Phenylketonuria |
| PMD | Pelizaeus-Merzbacher disease |
| PMN | Polymorphonuclear neutrophil leukocytes |
| PNET | Primitive neuroectodermal tumor |
| PNF | Peripheral neurofibromatosis |
| PNS | Peripheral nervous system |
| PO | By mouth |
| PP | Perfusion pressure |
| SAH | Subarachnoid hemorrhage |
| SCI | Spinal cord injury |
| SD | Standard deviation |
| SED | Spondyloepiphyseal dysplasia |
| SIADH | Syndrome of inappropriate antidiuretic hormone |
| SPECT | Single photon emission computed tomography |
| SPR | Selective posterior rhizotomy |
| SSEP | Somatosensory evoked potentials |
| ST-MCAA | Superficial temporal–middle cerebral artery anastomosis |
| $T_3$ | Triiodothyronine |
| $T_4$ | Thyroxine |
| TB | Tuberculosis |
| TS | Tuberous sclerosis |
| TSH | Thyroid-stimulating hormone |
| US | Ultrasound |
| VER | Visual evoked response |
| VL | von Hippel-Lindau disease |
| VSD | Ventricular septal defect |
| WBC | White blood cell |
| WISC-R | Wechsler Intelligence Scale for Children (Revised) |
| WPPSI | Wechsler Preschool and Primary Scale of Intelligence |

# Handbook of
# Pediatric Neurology
# and Neurosurgery

Notice

The indications and dosages of all drugs in this book have been recommended in the medical literature and conform to the practices of the general community. The medications described do not necessarily have specific approval by the Food and Drug Administration for use in the diseases and dosages for which they are recommended. The package insert for each drug should be consulted for use and dosage as approved by the FDA. Because standards for usage change, it is advisable to keep abreast of revised recommendations, particularly those concerning new drugs.

# Embryology

A variety of factors can contribute to abnormal development of the CNS. Environmental, maternal, and genetic factors and combinations of these may adversely affect the developing fetus. Environmental factors consist of such things as exposure to radiation and toxins. Maternal factors are such things as ingestion of drugs, metabolic abnormalities, and hemodynamic alterations. In most cases the specific causes are not known.

## I. NORMAL DEVELOPMENT
### A. Neural tube formation
1. **Primary neurulation (3–4 weeks' gestation).** This is the process of neural tube formation, except the most caudal portions. The neural plate initially develops on the dorsal aspect of the embryo as a plate of tissue differentiating from the ectoderm of the trilaminar embryonic disc. The proliferation of neuroectoderm to form a neural plate is induced by the underlying notochord. The neural plate then invaginates, folds, and fuses in the midline. The process of fusion begins in the region of the lower medulla and proceeds rostrally and caudally. The anterior neuropore closes at about 24 days and the posterior neuropore at 26 days. The posterior neuropore is at the L1–L2 level. More caudal segments are formed through a different process. After closure the neural tube separates from the surface ectoderm. The surface ectoderm differentiates into the epidermis of the skin. Some surrounding ectoderm cells at the crest of the neural fold differentiate into neural crest cells that go on to form the sensory ganglia of the spinal nerves, cranial nerves V, VII, IX, and X, and the autonomic nervous system, as well as the Schwann cells, pia mater, arachnoid, and other non-neural tissues. The surrounding mesoderm develops into dura mater and vertebrae.
2. **Secondary neurulation (4–7 weeks' gestation).** The formation of the lower lumbar, sacral, and coccygeal portions of the neural tube are formed by canalization and retrogressive differentiation. The **caudal cell mass**, a group of undifferentiated cells at the caudal end of the neural tube, develops vacuoles. These vacuoles merge together and expand, ultimately meeting the central canal of the rostral cord and causing elongation of the neural tube in a process called **canalization**. Overlapping with canalization, the process of **retrogressive differentiation** of the caudal cell mass takes place. In this process the filum terminale, conus medullaris, and ventriculus terminalis are formed. The conus medullaris initially rests in the coccygeal region and appears to ascend as the spine grows more rapidly than the cord. At birth the conus is usually at the caudal level of L2–L3 and by 3 months of age it is at L1–L2, where it remains.
### B. Formation of the vertebral column
1. Somites arise from the paraxial mesoderm beginning

around 20 days of gestation. After formation, the ventral and medial walls of the somites separate into sclerotomal cells. Masses of these cells are referred to as **sclerotomes**.

2. During the fourth week of gestation, cells from the paired sclerotomes on either side of the notochord fuse in the midline to surround the notochord. Some of these cells give rise to the intervertebral disc and others form the mesenchymal centrum of the vertebrae. Each vertebral body is formed by the caudal and cranial halves of adjacent sclerotomes, with the notochord ultimately involuting. Between each vertebra, the notochord forms the nucleus pulposus, around which the annulus fibrosus develops to form the intervertebral disc.

3. The vertebral arch is formed by sclerotomes surrounding the developing neural tube.

4. In the sixth week of gestation, chondrification centers arise in the centrum and the arch.

5. Two primary ossification centers develop at 7 weeks' gestation. They are located in the centrum of the vertebrae and ultimately fuse. Once fused, ossification centers develop in each half of the vertebral arch.

6. At birth, the vertebrae are composed of three bony segments connected by cartilage.

7. The caudal spinal column is formed as the caudal cell mass (notochord, mesoderm, and neuroectoderm) forms somites, which develop into the sacral, coccygeal, and tail vertebrae. With retrogressive differentiation, the tail is lost.

## C. Formation of the brain

### 1. Gestational week 4

a. After closure of the anterior neuropore, the three primary brain vesicles are formed: **prosencephalon** (forebrain), **mesencephalon** (midbrain), and the **rhombencephalon** (hindbrain).

b. Rapid growth and flexion occurs. Midbrain flexure develops in the midbrain region and cervical flexure between the midbrain and the spinal cord.

### 2. Gestational week 5

a. The forebrain divides into two vesicles: the **telencephalon** and the **diencephalon**. The cavities within the developing brain are the future ventricular system and remain contiguous with the central canal of the spinal cord for much of fetal development.

b. Disproportionate growth in the hindbrain produces the ventrally convex **pontine flexure** which divides the **rhombencephalon** into the **myelencephalon** (medulla) and **metencephalon** (pons and cerebellum).

### 3. Myelencephalon

a. The rostral portion, because of the pontine flexure, is wide and flat. The roof becomes thin, and the future site of part of the fourth ventricle becomes rhomboid-shaped. On the lateral aspects, the alar (sensory) plates are pushed laterally to the basal (motor) plates such that the motor nuclei develop medial to the sensory nuclei. At the time of birth the obex becomes the end of the ventricular system as proliferation of the spinal cord cells causes obliteration of the central canal.

   b. The caudal aspect resembles the spinal cord except that dorsally the neuroblasts migrate to form the gracile and cuneate nuclei. Located ventrally in the medulla are the pyramids, which are composed of the descending corticospinal fibers.

**4. Metencephalon**

   a. The pons, cerebellum, and rostral portion of the fourth ventricle develop from the metencephalon.

   b. The dorsal aspects of the alar plates develop paired bilateral thickenings (rhombic lips) that fuse in the midline at 8 weeks and ultimately develop into the cerebellum.

**5. Choroid Plexus**

   a. The thin ependymal roof of the fourth ventricle and the mesenchymal-derived pia mater form the **tela choroidea**.

   b. With proliferation of the vascular pia mater, the tela-choroidea invaginates into the fourth ventricle and differentiates into the choroid plexus. A total of four choroid plexuses are formed in this manner (the roof of the third ventricle, bilateral lateral ventricles, and fourth ventricle).

   c. The foramina of Luschka and the foramen of Magendie perforate at approximately 9 weeks' gestation.

   d. Also at 9 weeks, the cells of the choroid plexus become secretory and begin to produce CSF.

**D. Formation of the skull**

   1. Mesenchyma surrounding the developing brain becomes the skull and the skeleton of the jaws.

   2. The skull base is composed of the occipital, ethmoid, sphenoid, and petrous temporal bones. It is formed by endochondral ossification. A cartilaginous base forms around the cranial end of the notochord and fuses with cartilage of the occipital somites. Through the process of endochondral ossification, the bones at the base of the skull are formed.

   3. The cranial vault (parietal and frontal bones) develops by a membranous process. Intramembranous ossification at the top and sides of the cranium forms the cranial vault. Sutures separate the bones of the vault and join together to form fontanelles. The sutures and the pliable nature of the membranous cranial vault allow molding to occur during birth.

**II. EMBRYOPATHIES.** The conditions listed below are significant surgical considerations and are further discussed in Chapter 8.

**A. Myelomeningocele.** The neural placode remains on the surface of the back through either a failure of primary neurulation or rupture of a closed neural tube.

**B. Dermal sinus tracts (cranial or spinal).** A persistent tract may remain at the site of closure of the caudal neuropore, the cranial neuropore, or anywhere in between. There is often an associated dimple. Dermal sinus tracts can be a cause of tethered cord or recurrent meningitis and should be repaired when discovered.

    **C. Lipomyelomeningocele.** Subcutaneous fat attached to the spinal cord can result from paraxial mesenchyma gaining access to the dorsal surface of neuroectoderm prior to fusion.

    **D. Diastematomyelia** is a division of the spinal cord into two hemicords. Postulated etiologies include the persistence of an accessory neurenteric canal that traverses the neural plate and notochord and causes abnormalities in one or both of them; and failure of the margins to touch each other at the time of primary fusion, instead curling inward to form two tubes.

    **E. Terminal myelocystocele** is an expansion of the distal end of the spinal cord into a terminal cyst. The spinal cord is usually tethered. It has been suggested that terminal myelocystocele develops as a result of CSF accumulation in the developing terminal ventricle, which disrupts the normal development of surrounding structures and causes spina bifida, meningocele, and tethered cord.

    **F. Embryonic deformation and caudal suppression syndromes.** This is a group of syndromes characterized by anomalies in the lower extremities, anorectal system, genitourinary organs, and lumbosacral spine. The embryology is a disturbance of the caudal mesodermal axis, abnormal caudal notochord and neuroectoderm development, and constriction of the embryo.

## III. SKELETAL MALFORMATIONS

    **A. Klippel-Feil syndrome** is a lack of segmentation in several segments of the cervical vertebral column. The syndrome is associated with a low hairline, restricted range of motion in the neck, and a short neck. Often there is an underlying Chiari malformation.

    **B. Hemivertebra** arises from failure of one of the chondrification centers to appear during vertebral development. Half of the vertebra fails to form. Hemivertebra often leads to scoliosis.

    **C. Spina bifida** may range from a relatively mild spina bifida occulta to total rachischisis (cleft of the vertebral column). These defects arise when the halves of the vertebral arch fail to fuse. The extent of involvement of the neural tube varies.

    **D. Cranioschisis (acrania)** is a failure of the anterior neuropore to close during the fourth gestational week with failure of cranial vault formation. Anencephaly usually results.

    **E. Craniosynostosis.** A variety of skull deformities arise from premature closure of the sutures (see Chapter 17 for further detail).

    **F. Craniovertebral junction anomalies** are present in 1% of newborns. They arise from abnormal bone development in the craniovertebral region and include atlantoaxial instability, foramen magnum abnormalities, axis and atlas malformations, and occipital bone malformations.

# Prenatal Diagnosis

Many abnormalities of the CNS can be detected in utero. The diagnostic tools available are blood tests, amniocentesis, and ultrasonography. The in utero diagnosis of neurological disorders allows for a comprehensive approach to management. An extensive review is beyond the scope of this text; however, some of the more common CNS anomalies and the diagnostic process for each are briefly discussed below. The prenatal diagnosis of genetically transmitted conditions is discussed elsewhere in the text.

## I. IN UTERO ABNORMALITIES
### A. Anencephaly
1. Elevated blood or amniotic fluid AFP levels.
2. Absence of the cranial vault on sonogram by 12–14 weeks' gestation.
3. Anencephaly can be confused with encephaloceles and amniotic band syndrome.

### B. Hydranencephaly
1. Craniomegaly.
2. Supratentorial hydrocephalus.
3. Hydranencephaly can be mistaken for maximal hydrocephalus or holoprosencephaly.

### C. Microcephaly
1. Biparietal diameter less than three standard deviations below the mean for gestational age and weight. The correct gestational age is essential for an accurate diagnosis.
2. Microcephaly can be misdiagnosed in cases of craniosynostosis where the biparietal diameter is decreased.

### D. Encephaloceles
1. Sacs with brain or CSF extending from the calvarium.
2. Hydrocephalus may be present.
3. Encephaloceles can develop in association with amniotic band syndrome.

### E. Myelomeningocele
1. Detected as a sac extending from the spine with abnormal bone formation.
2. Absence of lower extremity movement may be noted at the time of sonography in high lumbar or thoracic lesions.

### F. Hydrocephalus
1. Early in pregnancy the diagnosis requires a series of sonograms that show progressive, abnormal ventricular enlargement.
2. With diagnosis, workup for a TORCH infection should be initiated.

### G. Dandy-Walker syndrome
1. A fluid-filled posterior fossa with or without associated supratentorial hydrocephalus.
2. An increased biparietal diameter is often noted.

## II. PRENATAL DIAGNOSIS OF MALFORMATIONS
### A. If an appropriate workup and diagnosis are accomplished early, the parents can make an informed decision to abort the fetus if they choose to.

    **B.** Allows adequate time for counseling and preparation regarding the detected defect.

    **C.** Enables the early development of a comprehensive management program.

        **1.** Discussion with the parents regarding diagnosis, prognosis, and options.

        **2.** Case discussion between the obstetrician, pediatrician, pediatric neurosurgeon, and pediatric surgeon.

        **3.** Decisions made regarding mode and timing of delivery to optimize outcome.

    **D.** In the future, may allow for in utero surgical intervention for some malformations.

## III. BLOOD TESTS

    **A.** Open neural tube defects cause an elevated AFP in maternal serum. Eighty percent of open myelomeningoceles and ninety percent of anencephalies can be detected.

    **B.** Elevated AFP occurs most commonly with twins. It also occurs with fetal demise. These can be readily assessed using sonography.

    **C.** AFP levels vary with gestational age and inaccurate gestational dates can be responsible for an elevated AFP.

    **D.** Other non-neurosurgical causes of elevated AFP include Turner's syndrome, missed abortion, omphalocele, gastrointestinal obstruction, and sacrococcygeal teratoma.

## IV. AMNIOCENTESIS

    **A.** Amniocentesis allows for the examination of amniotic fluid to detect chromosomal anomalies, metabolic disorders, and NTDs.

    **B.** Amniocentesis should be performed prior to 18 weeks' gestation.

    **C.** It is indicated in cases of unexplained increased AFP.

    **D.** Amniotic AFP analysis and acetylcholinesterase gel electrophoresis can be combined to detect NTD.

## V. PRENATAL ULTRASOUND

    **A.** Ultrasonography is becoming increasingly used in obstetrical practice. This has led to an increase in the incidental discovery of fetal abnormalities.

    **B.** It should be used for screening in cases where there is a history of NTD or with advanced maternal age, when there is a higher risk of fetal malformations.

    **C.** It is important that an experienced physician perform the ultrasound to ensure appropriate diagnosis.

# Neurological Examination of the Premature Infant, Newborn, and Child

The neurological evaluation of children includes an assessment of the gestational period, delivery, postnatal medical history, parental medical history, and physical examination. The CNS continues to develop after birth and in fact does not reach maturity until about age seven. Therefore the neurological examination of children is unique. Much of the exam is based primarily on observation. Manipulation yields further information about tone, muscle strength, deep tendon reflexes, and superficial sensation. Testing of brainstem and spinal reflexes can then be performed. As children move toward adolescence the examination approximates that of the adult.

## I. PREMATURE INFANT

A. The neonatal neurological evaluation changes as the CNS matures. It is essential to ascertain the gestational age of the neonate for several reasons. The first and most obvious reason is to determine whether the examination is normal or abnormal. The second is to help determine the most likely pathophysiological process causing the abnormality, because certain disorders are related to gestational age. Tables 3-1 and 3-2 list some guidelines that are helpful in distinguishing the premature infant from the small-for-gestational-age infant.

B. More than 35,000 infants weighing less than 1 kilogram are born in the United States each year. Most of these infants survive with aggressive medical attention.

C. The most common neurological sequelae of prematurity are seizures and intraventricular hemorrhage (IVH). Hydrocephalus develops in 20–50% of cases of IVH.

D. The daily measurement of head circumference and examination of the fontanelle and sutures, along with routine cranial sonography, are appropriate surveillance.

1. The average rate of head growth for the first 3 months in a sick premature infant is 0.25 cm/week.

2. Healthy premature infants can be expected to have an increase in head circumference of 1.1 cm / week for the first 2 months, and then 0.5 cm / week for the third and fourth months.

3. Head circumference charts designed specifically for the premature infant are available (see Appendix).

E. Observation

1. The premature infant should be observed approximately 1 hour prior to a feeding to assess the level of alertness.

   a. Infants of 28 weeks' gestation often need stimulation in order to be aroused.

   b. Premature infants sleep 80–85% of the time, as compared with term infants, who sleep 60% of the time.

2. Lower gestational age infants tend to stretch in an unco-

**Table 3-1. Characteristics helpful in determining gestational age**

| External characteristics | 28 weeks | 34 weeks | 40 weeks |
|---|---|---|---|
| Ear cartilage | Pinna soft, folded | Pinna harder, maintains form after folding | Thin cartilage resumes shape after folding |
| Skin | Thin, clear | Pink, some abdominal vessels | Pale, few blood vessels |
| Sole creases | None | Two: anterior, transverse | Anterior 2/3 of sole |
| Breast tissue | None | 2 mm | 4 mm |
| Genitalia | | | |
| Male | Testes undescended | Palpable, high in canal, few scrotal rugae | Testes descended, scrotum with rugae |
| Female | Labia spread, large clitoris | Labia majora over labia minora | Labia almost covers clitoris |

**Table 3-2. Reflexes and their age of appearance**

| Reflex | Age absent | Age present |
|---|---|---|
| Pupillary reflex | <29 weeks | >31 weeks |
| Glabellar tap reflex | <32 weeks | >34 weeks |
| Head turning to light | <32 weeks | >36 weeks |
| Neck righting reflex | <34 weeks | >37 weeks |

ordinated, generalized fashion with frequent episodes of tremulousness and clonic movements.

  3. Beyond 32 weeks' gestation movements become more localized and coordinated.

**F. Cranial nerves**

  1. Prior to 36 weeks' gestation an infant will not turn toward a light stimulus. With a very strong light stimulus a premature infant may exhibit eye closure.

  2. The pupillary light reflex is absent prior to 29 weeks; it is not reliably present until after 31 weeks.

  3. Oculocephalic reflexes cannot be elicited until approximately 36 weeks' gestation, at which point infants are able to fixate on a light source. The loss of oculocephalic reflexes (i.e., the presence of "doll's eyes") beyond about 36 weeks is considered pathological.

  4. Vocalization in the premature infant is present, but difficult to elicit. When a cry is heard it is weak and short in duration.

**G. Motor**

  1. The motor responses are particularly useful in distinguishing the small-for-gestational-age infant from the premature infant.

  2. A 28-week premature infant is essentially flaccid. When held with the palm of the hand supporting the abdomen a premature infant will hang loosely without extension of the head, extremities, or spine.

  3. Maturity of motor development progresses in a caudocephalic direction.

     a. Infants at 34 weeks maintain the legs in a frog-leg position with persistent hypotonia and extension of the upper extremities.

     b. By 38 weeks the infant should be flexor in all four extremities.

  4. Responses to limb manipulation, righting, and postural reactions.

     a. The **scarf sign** is demonstrated by drawing the arm medially across the chest toward the opposite shoulder. The elbow reaches the opposite shoulder in the premature infant, but will not cross midline as the infant approaches term.

     b. Similarly, the heels can be placed next to the ears by flexing the legs to the head in the premature infant.

     c. A 28-week infant remains essentially flaccid. By 34 weeks there is some supporting response, and by 38 weeks this response is well developed.

     d. Prior to 30 weeks the head is not supported at all. As the head extensors and flexors develop, this slowly improves, and by 38 weeks the head will briefly follow the trunk, although it cannot be supported in the upright position.

**H. Reflexes**

  1. **Rooting** is weak at 28 weeks and has a long latency. By 34 weeks this reflex is fully developed.

  2. **Startle reflex** (Moro's reflex). At 28 weeks this reflex is only partially developed and lacks the adductor phase of the response. By 38 weeks the full reflex can be elicited.

    **3. Crossed-extension reflex.** When rubbing the sole of one foot with the leg in extension, the opposite leg will flex and withdraw and then extend while spreading the toes. This is not observed until 36 weeks.

    **4. Stepping.** The stepping response is absent in the 28-week infant. By 32 to 34 weeks stepping appears as toe walking. By term this will develop to a heel-toe response.

    **5. Sucking.** In the 28-week infant the sucking response is weak. By 34 weeks this response is complete.

## II. INFANTS AND CHILDREN

### A. Observation

1. With the infant in the arms of a parent, facial expression, extraocular movement, limb movement, and level of alertness should be noted.
2. Birth marks, epicanthal folds, unusual palpebral fissures, low-set ears, telangiectases, hemangiomas, ear tags, simian creases, and webbing suggest a variety of syndromes.
3. Head shape should be evaluated. Direct head circumference measurement plotted on a head circumference chart is essential (see Appendix).
4. Note the size and feel of the anterior fontanelle.
5. Developmental milestones can be observed. It is important to note that there can be significant "normal" variation in the attainment of milestones. A listing of some of the major developmental milestones is found in Table 3-3.

### B. Cranial nerves

1. **CN I.** Behavioral response to simple odors.
2. **CN II.** Movement of an object through all visual fields, assessment of pupillary response.
3. **CN III, IV, VI.** Visual tracking of an object.
4. **CN V.** Corneal reflex and history of chewing.
5. **CN VII.** Facial expressions.
6. **CN VIII.** Response to noises or a tuning fork.
7. **CN IX, X.** Quality of cry, gag reflex, history of feeding.
8. **CN XI.** Head movement.
9. **CN XII.** Tongue symmetry.

### C. Motor

1. Limb movement, symmetry, and spontaneity.
2. Assessment of muscle bulk and tone.
3. Limb posture at rest.
4. Response of muscles to passive stretch.
5. Infant's handling of objects presented to each hand individually. Hand preference does not develop prior to 18 months; if a preference is noted prior to this it may point to an underlying weakness or spasticity.
6. The reaching response of each arm as objects are presented to evaluate arm abduction and adduction.
7. Range of motion in the joints with passive movement.
8. Pull the infant by the hands to a sitting position. The head should not lag behind the arms after 5 months of age.

### D. Reflexes

1. DTRs may be absent on the first day of life.
2. Plantar reflexes are normally flexor in the newborn; however, withdrawal reflexes are common. Extensor responses suggest brainstem or spinal cord injury.

**Table 3-3. Developmental milestones**

| Age | Developmental milestones |
| --- | --- |
| 1 month | Raises head slightly from prone<br>Follows objects to midline<br>Tight grasp, hand fisted at rest<br>Alerts to sounds |
| 2 months | Lifts chest off table<br>Follows objects past midline<br>Social smile<br>Startles to loud noises |
| 3 months | Supports on forearms in prone position<br>Holds head position<br>Hands open at rest<br>Fixes and follows fully in all directions<br>Smiles and vocalizes<br>Laughs<br>Reaches for objects |
| 4 months | Rolls front to back<br>Sits when propped up<br>Reaches for objects and brings them to mouth<br>Orients to voice |
| 5 months | Lifts head while supine<br>No head lag<br>Babbles<br>Orients to bell |
| 6 months | Sits well without support<br>Puts feet in mouth while supine<br>Transfers objects between hands<br>Localizes sounds |
| 7 months | Stands briefly without support<br>Bangs objects on table<br>Says dada/mama |
| 9 months | Creeps, crawls, and cruises<br>Pulls to a stand<br>Uses a pincer grasp<br>Understands "no"<br>Waves "bye-bye" |
| 12 months | Walks alone<br>Throws objects<br>Uses 2 words other than dada/mama<br>Imitates actions |
| 15 months | Creeps up stairs<br>Walks backward |

**Table 3-3.** (continued)

| Age | Developmental milestones |
| --- | --- |
| | Builds a tower of 2 blocks |
| | Uses 4–6 words |
| 18 months | Runs |
| | Feeds self |
| | Imitates parents in tasks |
| 21 months | Walks up stairs |
| | Builds a tower of 5 blocks |
| | Uses 2-word combinations |
| 24 months | Walks up and down stairs |
| | Removes clothes |
| | Uses pronouns |

   **3.** Ankle clonus is normally present prior to 2 months of age.
   **4.** Following is a list of primitive reflexes; the age at which they are usually extinguished is in parentheses.
      **a.** Adductor spread of knee jerk (7–8 months).
      **b.** Moro's (5–6 months).
      **c.** Palmar grasp (6 months).
      **d.** Plantar grasp (10 months).
      **e.** Tonic neck response (6 months).
   **5.** Parachute response may be elicited in an infant 9 months or older, even in visually impaired or blind children.
   **6.** Anal wink, if absent, suggests spinal cord abnormality.
### III. OLDER CHILDREN
   **A. Observation**
      **1.** Listening to the child speak allows for the detection of dysphagia or dysphonia.
      **2.** Abnormal ocular movement, nystagmus, facial asymmetry, ptosis, lip smacking, staring spells, and abnormal motor movements can readily be observed.
      **3.** Interaction with parents should be noted as a clue to attention span and behavioral problems.
      **4.** Milestones for older children include jumping in place (36 months) and hopping on one foot (48 months).
   **B. Cranial nerves**
      **1.** The older the child becomes, the more "routine" the cranial nerve examination becomes. However, early on, special effort is required to do a thorough examination.
      **2. CN I.** While not commonly involved in childhood, a simple presentation of scents like peppermint or cloves should produce a behavioral response.
      **3. CN II**
         **a.** Gross vision can be tested with object naming prior to 4 years of age. An E chart can be used in the years prior to

visual recognition of the alphabet.

**b.** Visual fields can be examined by wiggling fingers in the visual field quadrants and having the child point to the wiggling finger.

**c.** Fundoscopic examination reveals the pale grayish optic disc of the young infant or the sharper yellow-orange disc of the older child and adult. Papilledema associated with increased intracranial pressure can be noted. In children with open sutures and a fontanelle, blurring of the nasal margin and absence of venous pulsations can be the only suggestion of increased pressure.

**d.** Pupillary constriction and dilatation to a light source should be noted.

**4. CN III, IV, VI.** Eye movement as an object is followed through the primary gazes.

**a.** Eye deviation in children is not uncommon and may occur unrelated to neurological disease. **Exophoria** and **esophoria**, which are not apparent on inspection, may be noted with a simple cover test. Tropias (**exotropia** and **esotropia**), on the other hand, are not controlled by cerebral integration of visual images, and may be noted on direct inspection.

**b.** With strabismus, a head tilt can develop to compensate. With lateral rectus palsies, the head is turned toward the side of the weak muscle. With weakness in the superior oblique or superior rectus, the head is tilted toward the shoulder opposite the weak muscle.

**c.** Weakness of the extraocular muscles may be related to impaired vision, ocular myopathy, pontine tumors, optic gliomas, other mass lesions, myasthenia gravis, ophthalmoplegic migraine, or increased intracranial pressure.

**d. Abnormal eye movements**

   **(1)** Eyes deviate away from an irritative cerebral hemispheric lesion (i.e., an epileptic focus).

   **(2)** Postictal eye movements are toward the irritative lesion.

   **(3)** In destructive cerebral hemispheric lesions (tumors) the eyes "look toward" the lesion, with a conjugate gaze palsy to the opposite side.

   **(4)** In brainstem lesions, the eyes "look away" from the lesion, with a conjugate gaze palsy toward the side of the lesion.

   **(5) Internuclear ophthalmoplegia** results from interruption of the MLF presenting with a medial rectus palsy with intact convergence. If the lesion is caudad in the MLF, nystagmus and a sixth nerve palsy can be noted. This is commonly seen in the setting of midbrain or pontine gliomas, demyelinating diseases, hemoglobinopathies, or brainstem vascular disease.

   **(6)** In the cerebral hemispheres, vertical conjugate movements and lateral conjugate movements are integrated. Therefore, cerebral lesions result in a defect that has both lateral and vertical components.

(7) In the brainstem, the vertical movements and lateral movements are mediated separately; vertical movements are mediated via the superior colliculi, and lateral movements through the pons. Lesions of the superior colliculi result in vertical movement dysfunction, whereas lesions of the pons produce disturbances of lateral gaze.

(8) **Internal ophthalmoplegia** is a fully dilated pupil that does not react to light or accommodation with normal extraocular muscle function. This suggests pathology in the third nerve or the ciliary ganglion. It can also occur in association with diabetes.

(9) **External ophthalmoplegia** is ptosis and complete paralysis of all the extraocular muscles with a normal pupillary response. This can be seen with tumors or vascular abnormalities of the brainstem, myasthenia gravis, Wernicke's disease, botulism, and lead intoxication.

e. **CN V.** Absence of a corneal reflex, atrophy of the muscles of mastication, and absence of a jaw jerk are signs of abnormal fifth nerve function.

f. **CN VI.** Facial asymmetry, tearing, salivation, and taste can be evaluated through standard techniques depending on the child's age.

g. **CN VIII.** Hearing can be tested by voice or tuning fork. Vestibular function can usually be assessed by history. Caloric responses should be reserved for patients with impaired responsiveness.

h. **CN IX, X.** Observation of the palate with phonation and assessment of the gag response. Vocalizations provide information about laryngeal function.

i. **CN XI.** Head movement normally, and against resistance, and palpation of the sternocleidomastoid and trapezius muscles.

j. **CN XII.** Examination of the tongue at rest and with movement. Attention to speech, chewing, and swallowing.

C. **Motor**
1. Muscle movement, tone, bulk, and strength through the testing of individual muscle groups with game playing as needed.
2. Observation of gait during normal walking, tandem gait, heel-and-toe walking, and hopping may uncover abnormalities.

D. **Reflexes** are tested in a routine fashion.

E. **Cerebellar function**
1. Performance of rapid alternating movements.
2. Head tilts are often present with cerebellar lesions or cerebellar tonsillar herniation.

F. **Sensation**
1. Touch with sharp and soft objects in a game-playing manner.
2. Vibration and position sense.
3. Observation of a histamine response (reddening of the

stroked skin where sensation is intact) in less cooperative children can be very useful.

4. Cortical sensory function can be assessed through naming objects placed in the hand, naming the part of the body touched with the eyes closed, recognizing letters and numbers drawn on the palm of the hand, and double simultaneous stimulation.

## G. Intellectual development

1. Observation during examination.
2. History from the parent to obtain information about grade in school, attendance of regular versus "special" classes, behavioral problems in school, favorite subjects and least favorite subjects, and actual academic scores. All of this information can provide important clues to intellectual delay.
3. Formal testing should be performed in patients with possible intellectual delay. Baseline testing should be considered in patients with conditions frequently associated with delay. Pre- and postoperative testing may be useful for identifying potential areas of difficulty so that they may be addressed with special education programs.

# Diagnostic Testing

A wide variety of diagnostic procedures is available for the workup and diagnosis of neurological disease. Some are widely available, and others are available only in specialized centers. Radiographic, neurophysiological, neuropsychological, and other examinations are discussed below.

**I.RADIOGRAPHIC INVESTIGATION.** Many radiographic investigations cannot be adequately performed on a moving child. In such cases, medications for sedation are necessary. Chloral hydrate (25–50 mg/kg PO or PR; maximum 1 g/dose) or pentobarbital sodium (2–6 mg/kg/day divided tid PO or IM; maximum 100 mg/dose). In some cases, general anesthesia may be required to safely perform adequate studies.
  **A. Plain radiography.** A complete discussion of the applications of plain radiography in clinical neuroscience would be extensive. Appropriate applications are discussed throughout the book in relevant sections. Despite the development of advanced imaging modalities, plain radiography remains a useful tool in the practice of clinical pediatric neuroscience. Craniosynostosis, skull fractures, and spinal bony anomalies can frequently be diagnosed by plain radiographic imaging.
  **B. Computed tomography**
    1.An imaging modality based on ionizing radiation which produces high resolution images displayed as anatomical slices. Images can be displayed in axial, sagittal, coronal, or reconstructed 3-D slices. Intravenous contrast administration enhances the visualization of tumors and other regions of blood-brain barrier breakdown.
    2.CT scan is indicated for the assessment of congenital CNS anomalies, tumors, cranial or spinal trauma, and infection. CT is superior to MRI for the evaluation of acute trauma and bony anomalies and for detection of calcification (i.e., in tumor or infection). It remains a shorter and less costly examination and is still somewhat more widely available than MRI.
  **C. Magnetic resonance imaging**
    1.MRI is based on imaging the variable behavior of hydrogen protons within tissue exposed to a strong magnetic field. Hydrogen atoms, which have a net positive charge, are found in abundance throughout the body. They normally spin and create a small magnetic field. When exposed to the magnetic field of an MRI machine (15,000–150,000 gauss), protons flip from a low to a high energy level in a process called **resonance**. Resonance is encouraged by pulses of radio frequency photons directed into the body. Between pulsations, the protons realign with the magnetic field and emit a signal that is converted into an image. The image produced is based on the spin-relaxation rates of the tissues. T1- and T2-weighted images are produced. Gadolinium administered intravenously enhances the recogni-

tion of pathology on T1-weighted images in the same fashion as contrast does with computed tomography.

2. Appropriate applications of MRI are discussed in relevant sections. In general, MRI provides excellent anatomical detail for the diagnosis of congenital CNS malformations and the evaluation of intracranial and intraspinal tumors. MRI is superior to CT in the visualization of the gray-white junction and as such is useful in the evaluation of demyelinating conditions. It is also indicated in the workup of intractable seizure disorders.

3. MR angiography is a software application that selectively images vessels and provides an image similar to an angiogram. While MR angiography is a useful technique, conventional angiography is currently superior in the evaluation of vascular malformations.

## D. MRI spectroscopy

1. This modality is not widely available. It has the capacity to measure high-energy phosphates (e.g., adenosine triphosphate), intracellular pH, and lactate production.

2. The primary applications have been in the investigation of cerebral ischemia and muscle disorders.

## E. Ultrasound

1. High-energy sound waves (5–10 megahertz) are projected into the body in periodic pulses from the surface of the skin using a transducer. These sound waves respond differentially to liquid and solid substances. Sound waves travel through sonolucent (liquid) substances and are reflected off solid substances. The returning echoes are converted into an electrical signal that is amplified and displayed as dots of light.

2. US has a variety of applications in the practice of clinical pediatric neuroscience. It is particularly appealing in that it is a portable modality that does not require the transport of critically ill infants.

   a. US is particularly useful in infants prior to closure of the anterior fontanelle. Premature infants can undergo serial US to assess for intraventricular hemorrhage and the development of hydrocephalus. It can be used as a screening tool for the evaluation of the intracranial contents of neonates. Of course, it does not have the resolution of CT or MRI, and these studies are often indicated in the setting of abnormal findings on US.

   b. US through spina bifida defects is useful in the evaluation of tethered cord and intraspinal pathology such as tumors, syringomyelia, and diastematomyelia.

   c. Intraoperative US is used for guidance in finding deep brain tumors and for the intraoperative imaging of spinal cord tumors, cysts, and syrinxes. It may also be useful during decompression of symptomatic ACMs as a means to localize the fourth ventricle and associated syringomyelia.

   d. Prenatal US is useful for the detection of congenital anomalies such as hydrocephalus, intracranial anomalies, and neural tube defects.

## F. Positron emission tomography

1. PET is an imaging technique which provides anatomical images based on functional or physiological data. This is accomplished by the administration (intravenous or inhaled) of positron-emitting radiolabeled compounds that are incorporated into biological processes. The activity of these radiolabeled organic compounds can be viewed by detectors which translate this information into anatomically based images.

2. Isotopes of oxygen, carbon, nitrogen, fluorine, and gallium have been used in PET scanning. FDG is commonly used for the measurement of local cerebral glucose metabolism. Similarly, the inhalation of $^{15}O_2$ allows for observation of local cerebral oxygen metabolism and the inhalation of $^{15}O$-labeled $CO_2$ can allow for measurement of local cerebral blood flow.

3. The short half-life of positron-emitting radioisotopes necessitates the production of these isotopes at the site of the PET scanner. Largely for this reason, PET scanning is still not widely available. It is, however, being used with increasing frequency. Current applications include preoperative evaluation in seizure surgery; distinguishing between tumor recurrence and radiation necrosis; evaluating the degree of tumor malignancy; and early diagnosis in HC. PET has also been used to investigate cerebral vascular disease in the hopes of better understanding the physiology of stroke and enabling the prediction of the potential for functional recovery. Its applications are being expanded to allow for the study of neurotransmitter receptor binding sites and as a guide to our understanding of the functional development of the human nervous system.

## G. Single photon emission computed tomography

1. SPECT allows for the three-dimensional imaging of the distribution of gamma-emitting radionuclides ($^{133}$Xe, $^{123}$I, $^{99m}$Tc). Currently, its primary use is in the investigation of cerebral perfusion. A radionuclide-labeled amine, $^{123}$I-N-isopropyl-p-iodoamphetamine, has been used in the study of cerebral ischemia.

2. SPECT can be used to measure regional cerebral blood flow. However, it is limited in that it does not quantify blood flow or yield information about cerebral metabolism. Its use is more widespread than PET, in large part because gamma-emitting radionuclides have a longer half-life and do not require on-site production.

3. Applications include the assessment of cerebral ischemia and the evaluation of intractable epilepsy.

## H. Myelography

1. Introduction of a nonionic contrast agent into the thecal sac by C1–C2 puncture or lumbar puncture. Plain radiography and CT follow instillation of the dye.

2. This technique is especially useful for the assessment of compressive entities (i.e., blocks due to metastatic diseases and tumors), tethered cord, diastematomyelia, and spinal anomalies, particularly craniocervical junction anomalies.

Delayed CT aids in the diagnosis of syringomyelia. However, MRI demonstrates this entity readily.

## I. Cerebral angiography

1. Serial radiographs are taken during the injection of contrast medium into the carotid and vertebral arteries.
2. Cerebral angiography is indicated for the study of vascular anomalies, cerebrovascular disease (vasculitis, stenosis, moya-moya, thrombosis), and traumatic vascular injury, and for defining the vascular supply to tumors.
3. Complications of angiography are uncommon but include stroke, hemorrhage, contrast anaphylaxis, and vascular damage.

## J. Specialized studies

### 1. Shunt studies

a. Instillation of a nonionic contrast agent into the shunt reservoir with follow-up skull x-rays at set intervals allows for observation of clearance of the dye as a means to assess shunt function.

b. The reservoir should be accessed using a small (27-gauge) needle. Up to 1 cc of spinal fluid is removed, and an equal volume of contrast instilled. Skull radiographs are taken immediately and then at 3-minute intervals up to 20 minutes. A functioning shunt should clear the contrast within 9–12 minutes. This study can alternatively be performed with the instillation of a radioisotope and use of a scintillation counter to observe clearance to the abdomen.

### 2. Cisternography

a. **Positive contrast cisternography** involves introduction of a contrast medium into the thecal sac by either a C1–C2 puncture or lumbar puncture. The patient is then placed in Trendelenburg's position to allow dye to flow into the posterior fossa. This technique improves visualization of posterior fossa anomalies such as ACM. MRI (when available) has eliminated the need for this technique. Positive contrast cisternography remains useful in the diagnosis and localization of CSF leaks. In these cases, dye can be observed collecting in the sinus through which CSF drains abnormally.

b. **Radioisotope cisternography** uses the same technique; however, a radioisotope is injected into the thecal sac. This technique is useful for the evaluation of CSF leaks.

## II. NEUROPHYSIOLOGICAL TESTING

### A. Electromyography

1. EMG in conjunction with NCV helps differentiate between disorders of the muscle, neuromuscular junction, peripheral nerve, plexus, root, and anterior horn cell. Information from these two studies helps determine the type of abnormality and may give clues to the severity of the abnormality as well.
2. EMG is performed by the insertion of a needle electrode into the muscle and the recording of action potentials with spontaneous, voluntary, and evoked muscle activity. The

number, duration, rate, and morphology of motor unit discharges aids in the determination of the site and type of pathology.

3. EMG is worthwhile in the diagnosis of neuromuscular disorders. It is also used intraoperatively during surgery on the cauda equina such as release of tethered spinal cord and selective posterior rhizotomy.

## B. Nerve conduction velocity

1. The conduction rate of motor or sensory nerves can be measured by applying brief electrical pulses to the nerve and recording and measuring distally in the same nerve. For motor nerves, the response can be measured in the muscle supplied.

2. NCV is often used in conjunction with EMG to evaluate muscular disorders. It is also used in the evaluation of peripheral nerve disorders to determine an axonal versus demyelinating disease. Other applications include the study of hereditary sensory and autonomic neuropathies, in the setting of peripheral nerve or plexus trauma and in the evaluation of entrapment neuropathies.

## C. Electroencephalography

1. A noninvasive method of investigating the functional activity of the brain by the placement of multiple electrodes over the scalp. It is a study which can be performed at the bedside, eliminating the need for transporting critically ill patients.

2. The EEG tracing is assessed for voltage, amplitude, frequency, waveform morphology, and distribution. Single tracings that are normal are of limited value. In many cases, continuous monitoring for 24 or more hours is necessary for diagnostic purposes. Characteristic EEG patterns associated with seizure disorders are discussed in Chapter 28.

3. Its primary application is the study of seizure disorders and paroxysmal disorders. It can also be used in the determination of brain death.

## D. Brain electrical activity mapping is a technique of mapping the electrical activity of the brain (EEG and evoked potential) using computers. It has been applied primarily in the diagnosis and assessment of children with learning disorders.

## E. Evoked potentials

### 1. Brainstem auditory evoked potentials

a. Potentials evoked by a series of clicks delivered to each ear sequentially reflect activity in the acoustic nerve (wave I), the cochlear nucleus (wave II), superior olivary nucleus (wave III), nuclei of the lateral lemniscus (wave IV), inferior colliculus (wave V), medial geniculate nucleus (wave VI), and the geniculocortical pathway (wave VII). The latencies of these waveforms aid in the localization of auditory dysfunction.

b. BAER is used for the assessment of brainstem function and the evaluation of hearing capacity in patients who cannot cooperate with routine audiometry investigations.

    **c.** BAER is useful in the evaluation of meningitis, brainstem tumors, and demyelinating disease. It is also appropriate in the neurophysiological assessment of coma.

**2. Visual evoked potentials**

    **a.** Visual stimulation can be performed by either flash or pattern. Flash stimuli are preferable for infants and uncooperative children.

    **b.** The VER is recorded from the occipital cortex. The amplitude, latency, and morphology of the VER provide information about the location and type of lesion.

    **c.** VER is helpful in the workup of lipidosis and demyelinating disease, and for the evaluation of vision in the premature infant.

**3. Somatosensory evoked potentials**

    **a.** SSEP is measured by the stimulation of a peripheral nerve and the recording of waveforms at various points along the somatosensory pathway (nerve, plexus, posterior columns of the spinal cord, dorsal column nuclei of the cervicomedullary junction, thalamus, and frontoparietal cortex). The common peroneal or tibial nerves and the median nerves are used most commonly.

    **b.** Latencies and interpeak latencies at specified points are calculated and compared with normal controls and the opposite side.

    **c.** SSEP is useful not only for diagnostic purposes (hereditary sensory and motor neuropathies, Friedreich's ataxia, plexus trauma) but also for intraoperative monitoring during spinal cord surgery.

**4. Motor evoked potentials**

    **a.** MEP is similar to SSEP. They provide assessment of the motor columns as opposed to the sensory tracts. The different types are based upon the site of stimulation.

    **b.** **Cortical** stimulating electrodes deliver a transosseous electrical shock to the motor cortex and a myogenic response is recorded in peripheral muscle groups. The disadvantages include the possibility of seizure activity and the unknown effect of repeated stimulation. Lower limb data are unreliable.

    **c.** **Spinal cord**. Stimulating the spinal cord and recording a myogenic response from the periphery. A laminectomy is needed to place the epidural electrode.

    **d.** **Neurogenic motor evoked potentials**. Stimulation electrodes are placed proximal to the site of surgery: the cortical bone of the spinous process during a posterior approach, or the disc during an anterior approach. Responses are recorded from the sciatic nerve either at the sciatic notch or popliteal fossa. The response elicited is neurogenic, not myogenic. Thus, intraoperative muscle relaxants can be used. Amplitude and latency are measured. Ischemia will first reduce amplitude with little change in latency. Mechanical insult first affecting the larger diameter fibers causes a significant prolongation of latency followed by a reduction in amplitude. NMEP is useful for spinal cord surgery and surgery on the thoracic aorta.

**F. Electronystagmography**
  1. The evaluation of eye movements at rest and with positional, rotational, and caloric stimulation. This test provides an assessment of the vestibular system.
  2. While used more commonly in adults with acoustic neuromas or Meniere's disease, ENG can be useful in evaluating children with vertigo.

## III. NEUROPSYCHOLOGICAL TESTING

**A.** Neurological disorders in infancy and childhood are frequently associated with impaired neurodevelopment. Early diagnosis of delayed or impaired development is the first step toward optimizing outcome. Appropriate screening tests should be routinely performed on all children. Serial testing is indicated in all conditions which may be associated with neurodevelopmental impairment. In cases where delay or impairment is identified, appropriate intervention should be made as quickly as possible.

**B.** The **Denver developmental screening test** provides a standardized assessment of gross motor, language, fine motor, and social skills from infancy to early childhood.

**C. Intelligence** is measured in preschoolers using the WPPSI and the Stanford-Binet Scale. School-age children can be evaluated with the WISC-R.

## IV. LUMBAR PUNCTURE. LP does not replace a shunt tap in the setting of a potential shunt infection.

**A. Contraindications**
  1. Funduscopic examination to rule out papilledema and thorough neurological evaluation to assess for focal neurological deficit should be performed prior to LP. If there is any concern for elevated ICP associated with a focal mass lesion, a CT scan should be performed prior to LP. In the setting of elevated ICP with a mass lesion, LP should not be performed because of the risk of herniation.
  2. LP should not be performed in the setting of lumbar infection, either subcutaneous or epidural, as there is a risk of introducing bacteria into the spinal fluid and causing meningitis.
  3. Coagulopathies and thrombocytopenia increase the risk of hemorrhage with LP. Correction of clotting factors should be verified before LP can be safely performed.

**B. Indications.** LP is indicated in the workup of CNS infection, hemorrhage, inflammation, degeneration, and demyelination. LP is therapeutic in the setting of intraventricular hemorrhage of prematurity and pseudotumor cerebri.

**C. Technique**
  1. LP can be performed with the patient in the lateral knee-to-chest position. In obese patients, the sitting position may be preferable.
  2. The region over the lower back is cleaned with Betadine solution and draped in a sterile fashion.
  3. After the injection of a local anesthetic, a 20- to 22-gauge needle is introduced in the midline between L5 and S1 in neonates, L4 and L5 in children, and L3 and L4 in older children to avoid injury to the conus medullaris. The needle

should be aimed toward the umbilicus to pass through the posterior-directed spinous processes.

4. The spinal needle should always be passed with the stylet in place and the bevel parallel to the long axis of the thecal sac. Upon puncture of the thecal sac, the stylet is removed and the **opening pressure** measured with a manometer.

5. Spinal fluid is allowed to drip spontaneously and collected in sterile containers. Closing pressures should be obtained after sample collection.

6. At the completion of the procedure, the stylet is reinserted and the needle removed. The puncture site is covered with a bandage.

## D. Cerebrospinal fluid examination

1. **Opening pressure.** The normal opening pressure in newborns is close to 100 mm $H_2O$ and in older children it may be up to 180 mm $H_2O$. These are notoriously unreliable parameters in infants and young children because most children are crying and struggling during the procedure, causing an artificially elevated reading.

2. **Appearance.** Normal spinal fluid is clear and colorless. Cloudy or xanthochromic fluid is not normal. CSF with more than 500 RBCs /$\mu$l appears grossly hemorrhagic.

3. **Routine studies** (see Table 4-1).

   a. **Tubes 1 and 4. Cell count and differential.** In an atraumatic tap there will be almost no cells present. With a traumatic tap the fluid may be grossly bloody or have increased erythrocytes on microscopic examination. An increasing or stable number of erythrocytes suggests subarachnoid blood; a decreasing red cell count suggests a traumatic tap. In general, there is one white cell increase per 700 erythrocytes. If **xanthochromia** is present, hemorrhage occurred at least 4 hours prior to LP.

Table 4-1. Normal CSF characteristics by age

| Feature | Neonate | Child |
|---|---|---|
| Pressure (mm $H_2O$) | 100 | <180 |
| WBC (cells/$\mu$l) | 5–32 | 3 |
| RBC (cells/$\mu$l) | 20–50 | 0 |
| Glucose (mg/dl) | 50–80 | 50–80 |
| Protein (mg/dl) | 90 | 15–35 |

**b. Tube 2. Glucose and protein.** A serum glucose should be obtained at the time of LP, as normal CSF glucose is two-thirds the serum glucose. CSF protein is elevated approximately 1 mg/1000 erythrocytes. CSF protein will also be elevated in pathological conditions such as tumors and compressive lesions.

**c. Tube 3. Microbiology studies** (aerobic, anaerobic ,and fungal; Gram's stains, India ink, and acid-fast preparations; and cultures as indicated).

4. **Specialized studies**

   **a. Cytology.** Used in the setting of brain tumors or systemic neoplastic processes with potential for CNS involvement.

   **b. Tumor markers.** ß-HCG, CEA, and AFP can be elevated with certain types of brain tumors and are further discussed in Chapter 24.

   **c. Oligoclonal bands and IgG.** Multiple sclerosis is associated with the presence of oligoclonal bands in 70% of cases. The CSF IgG index is usually increased.

   **d. Viral studies**

   **e. Serologic studies**

E. **Complications**

   1. Headache is the most common complication. This is usually positional in nature with symptoms on standing or sitting and relief with assuming the horizontal position. Treatment with bedrest for 24 hours is usually curative. In some cases, a blood patch may be required.

   2. Other complications occur uncommonly and include hemorrhage, backache, and damage to nerve roots. LP-related dermoid or epidermoid tumors are extremely rare.

# Chromosomal and Toxic Anomalies

Approximately 3% of newborns are affected by some form of birth defect. Over 500 recognizable syndromes with CNS involvement have been identified. Of these, roughly one third have a known genetic component. Anomalies of the larger autosomes tend to be associated with more severe anomalies than those affecting smaller autosomes. Most abnormalities of the autosomes are associated with hypotonia. Major duplications or deficiencies in autosomes and anomalies of large autosomes are usually lethal. In general, anomalies affecting the sex chromosomes have less abnormalities than those affecting the autosomes. Reviewed in this chapter are the more commonly seen chromosomal anomalies with an emphasis on the neurological sequelae. Also included are the toxic anomalies, fetal alcohol syndrome and fetal valproate syndrome.

**I. DYSMORPHOLOGY.** There are a number of features which, if noted singly or in groups, suggest the possibility of an underlying chromosomal anomaly. Following are some indications for chromosomal analysis**.**
   **A. Clinical suspicion** of an autosome or sex chromosome syndrome. Below are minor and major features found with anomalies. It should be noted that some of these are found in normal patients and, in and of themselves, do not mean a chromosomal anomaly is present. Patients with several of these findings should be considered for chromosomal analysis.
      **1.** Hyper-/hypotelorism.
      **2.** High nasal bridge.
      **3.** Small, low-set ears.
      **4.** Webbed neck.
      **5.** Occipital scalp defect.
      **6.** Small mouth.
      **7.** Small mandible.
      **8.** Microphthalmia.
      **9.** Low-set thumbs.
      **10.** Overlapping fingers.
      **11.** Polydactyly, syndactyly.
      **12.** Rocker-bottom feet.
      **13.** Polycystic kidney.
      **14.** Ambiguous genitalia.
      **15.** Abnormal dermatoglyphics.
   **B.** Mental retardation of unknown etiology or in the setting of several minor, or two or more major, congenital anomalies.
   **C.** Microcephaly without a history of perinatal insult.
   **D.** A family history of recurring stillbirths or neonatal deaths.
   **E.** The occurrence of a new, dominantly inherited syndrome.
**II. AUTOSOMAL ABNORMALITIES**
   **A. Down syndrome**
      **1.** Trisomy 21.
         **a.** Ninety percent of cases are due to a pure trisomy of chromosome 21.

    **b.** One to five percent involve a translocation between chromosome 21 and various other chromosomes.

    **c.** Mosaics with a small percentage (about 2%) of normal cells.

**2.** Down syndrome is the most common autosomal anomaly, with an incidence of 1:750 live births with a slight male predominance. There is a strong relationship between maternal age and the incidence of Down syndrome. With a maternal age of less than 20 the incidence is 1:2500 and with a maternal age of 45 or greater the incidence increases to 1:55.

**3. General features.** Diagnosis can be made with the presence of eight or more characteristic clinical findings.

    **a. HEENT.** Flattened facies (mongoloid), epicanthal folds, obliquely oriented eyes, dysplastic ears, Brushfield's spots (fibrous tissue deposits visible in the periphery of the iris), arched or cleft palate, and flattened occiput.

    **b. Skin and skeletal abnormalities.** Xeroderma and chronic hyperkeratotic lichenification, dysplastic pelvis, bony abnormalities of digits and middle ear bones, palmar simian creases, short limbs, club feet, syndactyly, hyperextensibility of limbs.

    **c. Cardiovascular.** Twenty to sixty percent have congenital heart disease (VSD, ASD, PDA).

    **d. GI abnormalities.** Duodenal stenosis or atresia, imperforate anus, congenital megacolon.

    **e. Hematology.** There is a 15-fold increase in the incidence of leukemia over the general population.

**4. Neurological features**

    **a. Clinical.** Hypotonia, mental retardation, increased incidence of infantile spasms, incomplete Moro's reflex, epilepsy (10%), and brachycephaly with late closure of the anterior fontanelle and metopic suture. Intelligence in the pure mosaic may approach normal.

    **b. Neuropathology.** Low normal brain weight, narrow, straight superior temporal gyrus (can be seen in normal patients), and rarely, holoprosencephaly, agenesis of the corpus callosum, or aqueductal stenosis.

    **c. Alzheimer's disease.** Patients with Down syndrome have a predisposition to develop Alzheimer's disease, often at an earlier age than the affected "normal" population.

**5. Course.** There is a shortened life expectancy, with one third of affected children dying in the first year of life and another half by age four. The remainder may survive to 60 years of age.

**6. Management**

    **a. Karyotyping** should be performed on all patients suspected of having Down syndrome. If a translocation type of anomaly is found, parental karyotypes should be performed, as this has consequences for future offspring (recurrence risk is 5–16% depending on the type of translocation).

    **b. Prenatal diagnosis** can be made beginning in the third month with studies of amniotic fluid or chorionic villi.

Mothers who are 35 or older, have a history of a prior Down syndrome birth, or who have a low maternal serum AFP are at higher risk of having a Down syndrome infant.

c. Correction of **heart malformation.**

d. **Hearing aids** placed at an early age may improve the delay in language ability.

e. **Cervical spine abnormalities,** primarily ligamentous laxity, are frequent and require appropriate management.

## B. Edwards' syndrome

1. Trisomy 18.

2. This syndrome is being recognized more commonly and the current incidence is approximately 1:3000–6500 births (3 females:1 male).

3. **General features.** Dolichocephalic skull with a prominent occiput and a mildly webbed neck. The ears are malformed and low-set. A characteristic overlap of digits (second over third and fifth over fourth) and retroflexible thumbs are present. Congenital heart disease, omphalocele, and horseshoe and polycystic kidneys are seen frequently.

4. **Neurological features.** CNS involvement is variable. Agenesis of the corpus callosum, gyral and lobar anomalies, neuronal heterotopias and dysplasia of the hippocampus, inferior olivary nuclei, and lateral geniculate have been noted. An increased incidence of meningomyelocele is also seen. Developmental and mental retardation with hypotonia followed by hypertonia are typical features.

## C. Patau's syndrome

1. Trisomy 13.

2. **Incidence.** 1:8000 live births with a male predominance.

3. **General features.** Microphthalmia, cleft lip and palate, and polydactyly are the typical triad, although one or all of these features may be absent with other anomalies present. These include low-set, malformed ears, dermal ridges of arches and whorls, cardiovascular anomalies, polycystic kidneys, undescended testes, and omphalocele.

4. **Neurological features.** Clinically these infants have developmental retardation, profound mental retardation, seizures (20–30%), hypotonia, feeding difficulties, and apnea. Variable expressions of arhinencephalia, such as absence of the olfactory bulbs and tracts (60–70%), monoventricle, and absent interhemispheric fissure, have been noted with trisomy 13. Holoprosencephaly is present in 17% of cases. Cerebellar heterotopias are seen frequently. There is also an increased incidence of neural tube defects.

5. **Course.** Half of these children die within the first month and only 20% survive to the second year. Five percent survive to 3 years of age.

## D. Cri-du-chat syndrome

1. Partial deletion of the short arm of chromosome 5 (5p-).

2. **Incidence.** 1:20,000–50,000 births. Up to 1% of profoundly retarded individuals have this syndrome.

3. **General features.** The name is derived from the infant's cry, which is described as being like a kitten's meow and is

thought to be due to abnormal laryngeal development. Other features include a downward slant of the palpebral fissures, epicanthal folds, moon-shaped facies, hypertelorism, simian crease, limb abnormalities, low birth weight with delayed physical growth, and large corneas. Scoliosis develops in 55–60% of cases.

4. **Neurological features.** Microcephaly, generalized hypotonia, and mental retardation (IQ <35).

5. Affected children may reach a developmental age of 6 with early intervention and schooling. Life span is decreased but survival into adulthood is common.

## III. SEX CHROMOSOME ABNORMALITIES

### A. Fragile-X syndrome

1. X-linked inheritance of a fragile site within the terminal region of the long arm of the X chromosome (Xq27–28). Among chromosomal anomalies it is second to Down syndrome as a cause of mental retardation. Among mentally retarded populations fragile-X syndrome is identified in nearly 6% of males and 0.3% of females.

2. Males with fragile-X syndrome are characterized by moderate to severe mental retardation, macro-orchidism (after puberty), a long face, prominent chin, large floppy ears, and connective tissue dysplasia. Sixteen percent of males with fragile-X syndrome exhibit autistic behavior. Motor and language development are delayed.

3. Females who are heterozygous for fragile-X have variable phenotypic expression and may have no apparent abnormalities. One third are mildly retarded and half have learning difficulties.

4. **Prenatal diagnosis** can be made from amniotic fluid cells or chorionic villi cultured in the absence of folic acid.

5. Behavior during childhood is characterized as hyperactive with emotional lability and some autistic characteristics. This improves somewhat with age. Life expectancy is normal.

6. **Treatment** with folic acid has not been shown to alter outcome.

### B. Klinefelter's syndrome

1. XXY.

2. **Incidence** of 1:500 liveborn males. Increased incidence with advanced maternal age. Incidence is 5.4:1000 in mental institutions. This chromosomal anomaly is not usually diagnosed until adulthood. Diagnosis can be made by buccal smear for X-chromatin.

3. **General features.** X-chromatin positive male with phenotypic male genitalia, hypogenitalism, hypogonadism, gynecomastia, lack of spermatogenesis, increased FSH, and behavioral abnormalities. During adolescence, scoliosis and vertebral collapse sometimes occur secondary to osteoporosis.

4. **Neurological features.** Cognitive disorders (delayed language, dyslexia, learning disorders), diminished IQ (96 compared with normal control of 105), intention tremor (up to 50%), and EEG abnormalities (spike and spike-wave) are typical findings.

**5.** Behavioral problems and decreased mental function become more apparent when the child enters school.

**6.** With age, inadequate virilization may become apparent. If inadequate testosterone levels are documented, replacement therapy with testosterone cypionate should be implemented starting at age 11–12. Life span is normal.

## C. XXX syndrome

**1.** 47XXX.

**2.** **Incidence.** 1–2:3000 live births. This is increased with advanced maternal age.

**3.** **General features.** Normal to mildly dysmorphic features. Widely spaced nipples, hypertelorism, and fertility problems.

**4.** **Neurological features.** Decreased IQ (90 compared with a normal control of 100) to severe mental retardation. Microcephaly in some cases.

## D. XYY syndrome

**1.** Extra Y chromosome (47XYY).

**2.** **Incidence** of 1:1000 newborn males. Not usually detected in childhood.

**3.** **General features.** Phenotypic males with mildly abnormal features, tall stature, impulsive behavior (often antisocial), prominent glabella, severe acne in adolescence, and large deciduous and permanent teeth.

**4.** **Neurological features** include poor motor coordination with relative weakness, intention tremor, dull mentation, decreased NCV, and lower alpha wave frequency on EEG. Fifty percent have educational difficulties.

**5.** While XYY syndrome is not often diagnosed in childhood, the behavioral disturbances and diminished intellectual function lead to an increase in institutionalization for delinquency. Fertility is not usually affected, and transmission of the abnormal karyotype is rare. Life span is normal.

## E. Turner's syndrome

**1.** 45XO.

**2.** **Incidence** of 1:5000 live births.

**3.** **General features.** Short stature, redundant skin at the nape of the neck, congenital lymphedema, broad chest with widely spaced nipples, ovarian dysgenesis with hypoplasia, cardiac abnormalities of the left ventricular outflow system, and renal anomalies. In adolescence affected females may have primary amenorrhea and delayed physical development.

**4.** **Neurological features.** Hearing impairment and impaired spatial ability are common. Mental retardation is not typical as previously thought.

**5.** The course is not well known, although a survivor to the age of 90 has been described.

**6.** Cyclic estrogen replacement should be started around puberty. Lifespan is normal in the absence of significant cardiovascular or renal anomalies. Mosaics with 45X/46XY have an increased incidence of gonadal neoplasia and should have gonads removed.

## IV. OTHER ANOMALIES
### A. Börjeson-Forssman-Lehmann syndrome
1. X-linked recessive.
2. **General features.** Obesity, narrow palpebral fissures, large ears, hypogonadism.
3. **Neurological features.** Seizures, severe mental retardation, and hypotonia.
4. Early development is marked by hypotonia and developmental delay. Speech is reduced to a few phrases. Life expectancy is normal.

### B. Cleidocranial dysplasia
1. Autosomal dominant with high penetrance but variable expression. One third of cases are new mutations.
2. **General features.** Aplasia of all or part of both clavicles resulting in abnormal shoulder movements. Additional features include a high, arched palate and delayed or failed eruption of teeth. Pelvic dysplasias, cervical ribs, and other skeletal malformations occur frequently.
3. **Neurological features.** Brachycephaly, delayed closure of fontanelles and sutures, wormian bones, syringomyelia, scoliosis, and vertebral malformations. Mentation is usually normal.
4. Life span is normal. Diagnosis is usually at birth by examination and radiographs.

### C. Cockayne's syndrome
1. Autosomal recessive.
2. **General features.** Cataracts, retinal degeneration, senile changes beginning in infancy, and photosensitivity of thin skin.
3. **Neurological features.** Intracranial calcifications, weakness, peripheral neuropathy, impaired hearing, and mental retardation.
4. Starting in late infancy, growth is retarded with loss of adipose tissue.

### D. Cornelia de Lange's syndrome
1. The majority of cases are thought to be sporadic. Some cases appear to have an autosomal dominant inheritance pattern.
2. **General features.** A weak, low-pitched cry in infancy, micromelia, downturned upper lip, synophrys (eyebrows grown together), and shortness of stature.
3. **Neurological features.** Mental retardation, initial hypertonicity, and seizures (20%).

### E. De Sanctis-Cacchione syndrome
1. Autosomal recessive transmission resulting in defective DNA repair.
2. **General features.** Xeroderma pigmentosa.
3. **Neurological features.** Microcephaly, seizures, mental retardation, variable spasticity, hypothalamic dysfunction, and cortical and cerebellar atrophy.
4. Life expectancy is reduced secondary to an increased incidence of malignancy and CNS dysfunction.

### F. Laurence-Moon-Biedl syndrome
1. Autosomal recessive.
2. **General features.** Obesity, hypogonadism, hypogenitalism, polydactyly, and retinitis pigmentosa.

      **3.Neurological features.** Mental retardation and progressive vision loss.

      **4.**Life expectancy is normal, but early death may occur due to renal or cardiac disease.

## G. Lowe syndrome

    **1.**Sex-linked recessive.

    **2. General features.** Glaucoma, cataracts, aminoaciduria, and organic aciduria.

    **3.Neurological features.** Choreoathetosis, hypotonia, mental retardation, and seizures.

    **4.**Development is markedly delayed.

    **5.**Treatment with sodium-potassium citrate corrects the acidosis and improves bone mineralization and growth rate.

## H. Meckel-Gruber syndrome

    **1.**Autosomal recessive inheritance.

    **2.General features.** Polydactyly and cystic dysplasia of the kidneys.

    **3.Neurological features.** Posterior encephalocele and microcephaly.

    **4.**Few patients survive longer than a few days or weeks.

## I. Miller-Dieker syndrome

    **1.**A defect of p13 on chromosome 17.

    **2.General features.** Upslanted palpebral fissures, small nose with upturned nares, and low-set ears.

    **3.Neurological features.** Microcephaly, mental retardation, hypotonia, opisthotonos, and seizures. Lissencephaly, heterotopias, small brainstem, and an absent or hypoplastic corpus callosum are anatomical features.

    **4.**Death usually occurs within the first 2 years.

## J. Prader-Willi syndrome

    **1.**Probable sporadic occurrence with some risk of inheritance. Nearly half of cases have been found to have a deletion in the q11–13 region of chromosome 15.

    **2.General features.** Obesity, small hands and feet, light hair and blue eyes, fair skin, and a small penis.

    **3.Neurological features.** Hypotonia, mental retardation, microcephaly, and seizures.

    **4.Course.** Often there is a history of decreased fetal movements. Hypotonia can be sufficiently severe in infancy to cause respiratory and gastrointestinal malfunction. This improves with age and a tendency toward obesity prevails. Testosterone therapy at adolescence should be considered.

## K. Rubenstein-Taybi syndrome

    **1.**Unknown etiology.

    **2.General features.** Slanted palpebral fissures, hypoplastic maxilla, and broad thumbs and toes.

    **3.Neurological features**. Absence of the corpus callosum, mental deficiency, vertebral anomalies, large anterior fontanelle, EEG abnormalities, and seizures.

    **4.**Feeding difficulties and recurrent respiratory infections in infancy are common.

## L. Schwartz-Jampel syndrome

    **1.**Autosomal recessive.

    **2.General features.** Blepharophimosis and joint limitation.

    **3.Neurological features.** Primary muscle disorder with

myotonia, muscular hypertrophy (50%), and normal to mildly impaired intellect.

4. The course is one of progressive myotonia with muscle wasting or hypertrophy.

**M. Sjogren-Larsson syndrome**

1. Autosomal recessive.
2. **General features.** Ichthyosis, obesity, and retinitis pigmentosa.
3. **Neurological features.** Mental retardation, spasticity, and, occasionally, seizures.

**N. Smith-Lemli-Opitz syndrome**

1. Autosomal recessive.
2. **General features.** Persistent vomiting, hypospadias, cryptorchidism, upturned nares, and ptosis.
3. **Neurological features.** Moderate to severe mental retardation, microcephaly, and seizures.

**O. X-linked hydrocephalus syndrome**

1. X-linked recessive.
2. **General features.** Hydrocephalus (aqueductal stenosis), mental retardation, cortical thumb.
3. **Neurological features.** Not all affected males have hydrocephalus.
4. Early shunting is the optimal treatment.

**P. Zellweger syndrome (cerebrohepatorenal syndrome)**

1. Autosomal recessive. It has been postulated that there is a defect in peroxisomal enzymes that play a role in lipid synthesis.
2. **General features.** Flat facies, high forehead, hepatomegaly, and camptodactyly.
3. **Neurological features.** Seizures, hypotonia, poor suck, and absent DTR. Pathologically, pachygyria, polymicrogyria, and myelination abnormalities have been noted.
4. Most of these infants die in the first year of life.

**V. TOXIC ANOMALIES**

**A. Fetal alcohol syndrome**

1. Alcohol is the most common fetal teratogen, affecting 1 in 1000 infants. As few as two drinks/day can have mild effects on the fetus (e.g., low birth weight). Consumption of 4–6 drinks/day can produce subtle clinical features, and 8–10 drinks/day results in severe fetal alcohol syndrome.
2. **General features.** Growth deficiency (starting in utero), short palpebral fissures, joint anomalies, and heart murmurs associated with ventricular and atrial septal defects.
3. **Neurological features.** Microcephaly, diminished IQ (50–80; mean 63), decreased fine motor function and eye-hand coordination, irritability, and hyperactivity. Less commonly, meningomyelocele, cervical vertebral anomalies, heterotopias, and hydrocephalus occur.
4. The severity of the syndrome is directly correlated with the degree of maternal alcohol consumption. Early on, infants are irritable. As children, they tend to be hyperactive and have profound intellectual compromise.

**B. Fetal valproate syndrome**

1. **Etiology.** Exposure to valproate in utero.

2. **General features.** Epicanthal folds connecting with an infraorbital crease, short nose with upturned nares, midface hypoplasia, small mouth, cleft lip and palate, and cardiovascular abnormalities.

3. **Neurological features.** Meningomyelocele and mental deficiency.

4. Similar findings may occur with in utero exposure to primidone, barbiturates, and hydantoins.

# Congenital Malformations of the Brain

Congenital malformations of the brain fall under several categories. The dysraphic lesions are discussed in Chapter 8. Included here are disorders involving failure of normal embryonic progression, including failures of cleavage, disorders of migration, sulcation, proliferation, and commissuration. Cystic lesions of the posterior fossa and supratentorial compartment as well as hydranencephaly are discussed.

## I. DISORDERS INVOLVING FAILURE TO CLEAVE

A. **Holoprosencephaly** is failure of the embryonic prosencephalon (forebrain) to cleave normally into two hemispheres. This may be a partial or complete defect. A variety of craniofacial malformations can be associated with this deformity. These include cyclopia (single, midline orbit), cebocephaly (one optic canal, absence of the nasal septum, and premaxilla), and ethmocephaly (absence of nasal bones, turbinates, ethmoid septum, and premaxilla). In general, the more severe the failure of the forebrain to divide, the more severe the craniofacial malformations. Holoprosencephaly can be associated with progressive hydrocephalus requiring treatment. The different types are described below.

1. **Alobar holoprosencephaly** is the presence of a monoventricular cerebrum without lobes or hemispheres. A posterior dysplastic membrane of cerebral mantle may be present. Olfactory bulbs and tracts are present. The malformed brain is typically small.

2. **Semilobar holoprosencephaly** represents partial differentiation of the prosencephalon with incomplete lobe formation. An interhemispheric fissure is present. The striate bodies are fused in the midline.

3. **Lobar holoprosencephaly** reveals well formed lobes and an interhemispheric fissure. Associated ocular abnormalities ranging from cyclopia to coloboma frequently occur.

## II. DISORDERS OF MIGRATION AND SULCATION

A. **Lissencephaly** (agyria) is characterized by the absence of cerebral convolutions, giving the brain a smooth appearance. A sylvian fissure is commonly present. This condition can occur bilaterally or unilaterally. The brain is typically small with some degree of ventriculomegaly.

B. **Pachygyria** is a less severe form of lissencephaly. While pachygyria and lissencephaly are often used interchangeably, this is not technically correct. In pachygyria there are usually some broad gyri lacking secondary gyri. As with lissencephaly, it can involve one or both hemispheres and the ventricles are usually large.

C. **Polymicrogyria** (micropolygyria) involves numerous pseudoconvolutions within the gyri, giving the brain a characteristic bossed appearance on the surface. It can be associated with cerebellar microgyria.

    **D. Neuronal heterotopia** involves impaired or arrested migration of neuroblasts resulting in abnormal accumulation of nerve cells in abnormal locations. They can appear as nodular masses along the ventricular walls or as diffuse, abnormal cells throughout the white matter.

## III. DISORDERS OF PROLIFERATION

    **A. Schizencephaly** is characterized by the presence of symmetrical, abnormal cavities or clefts that can be covered by a pia-arachnoid membrane or normal dura. Hydrocephalus can be present. This disorder is usually associated with severe mental retardation, seizure disorders, and spastic quadriplegia.

    **B. Micrencephaly** (small brain) is defined as an adult brain weighing less than 900 g. Microcephaly is usually present. It is frequently the result of anoxia or infection occurring perinatally and as such is not a true malformation. A recessively inherited familial micrencephaly occurs with brain weights of 500–600 g.

    **C. Megalencephaly** (large brain) is defined as an adult brain weighing 1600–2850 g. This is associated with epilepsy and mental retardation. It also occurs in those with normal and above normal intelligence.

    **D. Hemimegalencephaly** is rarer and can occur with hemihypertrophy. It may be the source of intractable seizures.

## IV. DISORDERS OF COMMISSURATION

    **A. Agenesis/hypogenesis of the corpus callosum** involves complete or partial absence of the corpus callosum. It often occurs in association with other malformations such as myelomeningocele, Dandy-Walker syndrome, ventricular septal defect, various somatic anomalies, and disorders of cleavage, migration, or sulcation. It can be clinically insignificant or associated with mental retardation and seizures.

    **B. Agenesis/hypoplasia of the septum pellucidum** often occurs in association with abnormalities of the corpus callosum.

## V. HYDRANENCEPHALY is the consequence of a perinatal lesion

resulting in absence of the cerebral hemispheres. A thin gliotic membrane can be present as a "cerebral mantle." The diencephalon, midbrain, pons, and medulla are preserved. The etiology of hydranencephaly is presumed to be bilateral cerebral necrosis as a result of bilateral internal carotid artery occlusion early in gestation. The occlusion is thought to be secondary to infection or compromise of the umbilical cord by amniotic tissue (amniotic bands). Obstruction of the CSF pathways causing progressive hydrocephalus may result in progressive macrocephaly. Placement of a shunt to facilitate nursing care is an option. Most patients with hydranencephaly die by 2 years of age.

## VI. DANDY-WALKER SYNDROME is a malformation involving

the posterior fossa structures with a cystic dilatation of the fourth ventricle and a hypoplastic or aplastic cerebellum. Atresia of the foramina of Magendie and Luschka can be present. Secondary stenosis of the aqueduct of Sylvius may be the cause of the associated hydrocephalus. Associated anomalies include agenesis of the corpus callosum, polydactylism, renal defects, spinal dysplasia, and neuronal heterotopia. Treatment involves CSF diversion of the ventricles, the cyst, or both.

## VII. ARACHNOID CYSTS

  A. Benign congenital anomalies composed of arachnoid-lined cavities usually filled with a clear, colorless fluid much like CSF.

  B. These cysts do not obviously communicate with the subarachnoid space or ventricular system. An unseen ball-valve type of communication may explain the progressive enlargement that is sometimes seen with these lesions.

  C. They occur (in order of frequency) in the Sylvian fissure, cerebellopontine angle, supracollicular area, vermian area, and other locations.

  D. Presentation is variable. Arachnoid cysts are often found incidentally on radiographs obtained for other reasons. They may or may not be associated with mass effect. If so, they can present with signs of increased ICP, headaches, seizures, focal neurological deficits, or mental retardation.

  E. Treatment of symptomatic arachnoid cysts involves craniotomy with marsupialization of the cyst or shunting or stenting of the cyst. Observing these lesions in the developing brain may not be in the best interest of the child because there is some evidence that they expand slowly over time. In many cases, when treated at an early age, the parenchyma expands after adequate decompression. Treatment should be individualized.

# Birth Injuries

Despite advances in obstetrical care, birth injuries remain a common problem. A variety of injuries to the central and peripheral nervous system occur at birth. These injuries range from the insignificant to the fatal. Some result in significant morbidity. Early diagnosis and prompt treatment are vital to optimize outcome. A variety of birth injuries and their management are discussed below.

## I. SKULL FRACTURES
- **A.** May be due to an intrauterine or delivery event.
- **B.** Most commonly birth-related depressed fractures are in the parietal or frontal region.
- **C.** **Ping-pong** fractures refer to depressed fractures without edema or bruising of the overlying skin secondary to pressure on the fetal cranium by the maternal sacral promontory. Ping-pong type fractures can also be seen as traumatic injuries in the early postnatal period when the bone is still thin and pliable.
- **D.** Surgical intervention may be necessary if the depression is significant (5 mm or more). Occasionally these will spontaneously reduce.

## II. BRACHIAL PLEXUS INJURIES
- **A.** Reported in large series to occur at about 2:1000 live births. Bilateral injuries are associated with breech presentation and occur in 8–23% of cases.
- **B.** The mechanism of injury is often mechanical traction separating the head from the shoulder during delivery.
- **C.** Risk factors for injury include breech presentation, forceps delivery, maternal diabetes, multiparity, large birth weight, shoulder dystocia, and prolonged second stage labor.
- **D.** Associated injuries include torticollis, facial nerve injury, clavicular fracture, and humerus fracture.
- **E.** Four basic types of injury are seen.
    - **1. Avulsion** results from the complete preganglionic disconnection of the root(s) from the spinal cord.
    - **2. Neurotemesis** is the postganglionic disconnection of the nerve. This injury has no potential for recovery.
    - **3. Axonotemesis** refers to disruption of the axon with an intact "nerve sheath," allowing for the potential for partial recovery.
    - **4. Neuropraxia** is a "bruise" of the nerve with axonal and neural elements intact, maintaining the potential for complete recovery.
- **F.** **Clinical presentation**
    - **1.** C5 and C6 are most commonly involved with the addition of C7 in some cases. A level will become evident within 6 weeks after birth.
    - **2.** Upper brachial plexus injuries (**Erb's palsy**) develop a "waiter's tip" posture of the upper extremity. The shoulder is adducted and internally rotated, the elbow extended, the forearm pronated, and the wrist and fingers flexed.

3. Isolated lower brachial plexus injuries are seen less commonly. **Klumpke's palsy** refers to a lesion limited to C8 and T1. Preganglionic injury at T1 is associated with Horner's syndrome and ptosis.

4. Complete lesions present with a flaccid limb, Horner's syndrome, and ptosis.

5. Associated injuries occur (see above).

G. **Management.** A multidisciplinary team composed of a pediatric neurosurgeon, orthopedic surgeon, and plastic surgeon, as well as a psychiatrist, physical medicine physician, neurologist, and physical and occupational therapists is ideal.

H. Extensive radiographic evaluation is required. Appropriate studies, with the likely abnormal findings in parentheses, are listed below.

1. Cervical spine (subluxation).

2. Chest (diaphragmatic paralysis, fractured clavicle).

3. Shoulder/arm (dislocation or fracture).

4. CT/myelography (pseudomeningoceles, failure to visualize a nerve in the root sleeve).

5. MRI (nerve root disruption, pseudomeningocele).

I. **Electrodiagnostic studies.** Evoked response, EMG, and nerve conduction (not accurate in the initial 2–4 weeks of life) can detect Wallerian degeneration or early renervation. The prognostic significance of these tests is debatable.

J. Eighty to ninety-five percent of infants with brachial plexus birth injuries will have complete functional recovery without treatment.

K. The sooner the recovery process begins, the more complete it is likely to be.

L. Infants without evidence of spontaneous recovery by 3 months of age have a poor prognosis without surgical intervention.

M. Infants with no evidence of renervation on electrodiagnostic studies or infants who do not achieve significant motor improvement by 3–4 months of age are considered surgical candidates.

N. Surgery should be performed at 4–6 months of age to ensure maximal recovery. Exploration with neurolysis, excision of a neuroma, or interpositional nerve grafts can be performed based on the type of injury.

O. Recovery of some function can be expected within the first 4 postoperative months.

## III. SPINAL CORD INJURIES

A. Several fetal positions are associated with SCI during birth. Sixty percent of SCI occur with breech presentation. Transverse lie and cephalic presentation requiring forceps extraction can result in SCI.

B. **Mechanism.** Traction applied to the shoulder or trunk stretches the spinal column and cord.

C. Most commonly, injury involves the upper cord, brainstem, or cervicothoracic junction.

D. At birth, affected infants have low Apgar scores with poor respiratory effort, reduced or absent movement of the extremities, poor feeding, and a weak cry.

E. These injuries can easily be mistaken for neuromuscular

disease.
**F.** Diagnosis can be made with MRI, CT, or myelography. Cord enlargement, hemorrhage, and disruption can be present.
**G.** Prognosis is poor. Mortality is in the range of 50%. Only 25% will make a reasonable recovery.

## IV. HEMORRHAGES

**A. Scalp (caput succedaneum).** Soft tissue injury or bleeding into the scalp is usually mild. More extensive hemorrhage can occur with vacuum extraction. Significant hemorrhage into the scalp can cause hemodynamic instability, disseminated intravascular coagulation, and even death. Treatment involves transfusion and correction of the associated coagulopathy. Application of a tight head dressing is not advised because skin necrosis may occur.

**B. Subdural/epidural hemorrhage.** Perinatal subdural or epidural hemorrhages usually present within hours after delivery. There can be associated skull fractures. The normal molding of the cranium during delivery, or the use of forceps, can produce these lesions. Infants present with seizures, respiratory distress, a bulging fontanelle, and focal neurological deficits. Serum and urine drug screening should be performed on the mother and infant, since maternal cocaine use can be an etiological factor in the development of intracranial hemorrhage.

**C. Tentorial tears** occur rarely. The most likely mechanism is normal cranial molding during delivery with increased venous congestion. Treatment is expectant. Hydrocephalus may develop because of subarachnoid blood. External drainage can avoid the need for permanent shunt placement.

**D. Subarachnoid hemorrhage** can result from normal molding during delivery. This is the most common cause of minor subarachnoid hemorrhage in infants. The major consequence of more severe hemorrhage is the possible delayed onset (several weeks or months after birth) of hydrocephalus.

**E. Germinal matrix hemorrhages** are not traumatic lesions. Refer to Chapter 10 for further detail.

# Dysraphism

A number of malformations are included under the term dysraphism. Those involving the spine are loosely referred to as spina bifida. They are all complex malformations that result from the abnormal development of the central nervous system axis.

**I. MYELOMENINGOCELE** is a congenital malformation resulting from the abnormal development of the neural tube manifested in varying degrees. It is a malformation that involves the entire central nervous system. At the level of the spine, there is a midline lesion that contains CSF, meninges, and spinal cord elements. The neural placode is identifiable on the surface. The bony canal is malformed and can have varying degrees of hemivertebrae, absent vertebrae, kyphosis, and missing or malformed laminae. Cephalad, the malformation includes hydrocephalus, ACM, and the potential for other cerebral anomalies such as agenesis of the corpus callosum and gyral abnormalities. Systemically, there are urological and orthopedic abnormalities. Myelomeningocele is the most complex congenital malformation of the central nervous system that is compatible with life.

- **A. Etiology.** A variety of environmental and genetic etiologies have been proposed for the development of NTD.
  - **1. Genetic transmission** is multifactorial. Having one child with an NTD increases the risk of having a second child with an NTD to 3–5%.
  - **2. Embryology.** A variety of theories have been proposed regarding the embryology of this condition. Essentially two theories regarding the mechanism of the defect exist.
    - **a. von Recklinghausen's theory** states that there is an initial failure to form the neural tube correctly.
    - **b. Gardner's theory** asserts that there is disruption of a previously formed neural tube.
- **B. Incidence**
  - **1.** Myelomeningocele occurs in 1–5: 1000 live births, based on geographical area. The highest incidence is found in some regions of Ireland.
  - **2.** Females are more commonly affected than males.
  - **3.** Caucasians have a higher incidence than blacks or Asians.
- **C.** Late complications should be checked for routinely. In all of these conditions the integrity of the shunt system must be assessed first.
  - **1. Tethered cord** can present with progressive neurological deficit. Change in sensation, motor function, bladder function, or gait, and the development of orthopedic deformities such as pes equinovarus or valgus, or scoliosis, are common findings. Back and leg pain or spasticity also suggest a tethered cord. This entity is discussed in detail in Chapter 9.
  - **2. Hydrocephalus and shunt malfunction** present with signs of increased intracranial pressure or insidious intel-

lectual decline.

3. **Arnold-Chiari malformation** is a complex hindbrain malformation. The presence of snoring, poor feeding, apnea, sleep disturbance, crowing, and change in upper extremity function suggest a symptomatic ACM. These symptoms may also herald the development of shunt malfunction. Integrity of the shunt system should always be assessed at the initial evaluation of ACM.

4. **Syringomyelia** is the accumulation of CSF within the spinal cord. This can result in the development of scoliosis, numbness or weakness in the hands and feet, and neck or back pain. It may develop secondary to shunt malfunction or ACM.

5. **Neoplasia** of the urinary and gastrointestinal systems is a potential risk in cases of myelomeningocele. Carcinoma of the urinary tract is increased due to chronic irritation from infection. Increased gastrointestinal carcinomas are also noted in paraplegic conditions. Increased exposure to diagnostic radiation is a contributing factor in both conditions. Routine stool guaiacs and urine cytology should be performed.

## II. OTHER FORMS OF SPINA BIFIDA

A. **Meningocele** refers to a midline, skin-covered cystic lesion composed of CSF, meninges, and skin. While ganglion cells have been identified pathologically within these lesions, the underlying spinal cord and cauda equina are usually normal. There can be a thickened filum terminale or tethered spinal cord. Meningocele occurs in only a small percentage of patients with spina bifida. Some of these patients will go on to develop hydrocephalus.

B. **Anterior sacral meningocele** occurs when there is communication between the retroperitoneal or infraperitoneal space and the spinal subarachnoid space through a defect in the anterior sacrum. The mass that develops is a fibrous connective tissue capsule filled with spinal fluid, and may contain some sacral nerve root elements. This defect is three times more common in females. It is much less common than either meningocele or myelomeningocele. It usually presents in adulthood. Similar abnormalities may occur at the lumbar and thoracic level.

C. **Lipomyelomeningocele** is characterized by a lipomatous mass, usually skin-covered, with extension of the mass to the spinal cord. As a rule, this is not associated with hydrocephalus.

D. **Myelocystocele** is an abnormal dilatation of the central canal in the terminal portion of the cord with a tether. It can occur in conjunction with myelomeningocele. Other associations include omphalocele and extrophy of the cloaca.

E. **Neurenteric cysts** are the result of a ventral dysraphic state with intraspinal cysts lined with the mucosa of the alimentary tract. They can occur in conjunction with a dorsal or ventral spina bifida. The most common location is in the cervical and upper thoracic region. In the past they were thought to be the result of a persistent neurenteric duct. However, the neurenteric duct takes on a coccygeal location with development. It is now thought that these lesions are related to a failure of separation of the endodermal elements of the foregut from the neuroectoderm. They may be isolated or occur in association with a variety of malformations such as holoprosencephaly, anencephaly, Klippel-Feil syndrome, and an assortment of spinal deformities.

## III. OCCULT DYSRAPHISM

**A. Spina bifida occulta** refers to the incomplete formation of the bony spine with or without neural involvement. It occurs in 20–30% of the population (3–4 times more often in females) and should raise the concern that there is an underlying abnormality such as a lipoma, dermoid cyst, diastematomyelia, or tethered cord. Cutaneous stigmata overlying the bony abnormality (hypertrichosis, skin color changes, pinpoint "sinus," subcutaneous fatty tissue, telangiectasia, or capillary hemangioma) suggest an underlying abnormality. Radiographs on newborns can be misleading because of incomplete ossification.

**B. Diastematomyelia (diplomyelia)** involves a congenital splitting of the spinal cord. This condition is often associated with a cartilaginous or bony spicule that goes between the separated portions of the spinal cord. This can cause a tether of the cord or mechanical or vascular compromise as activity and growth occur. A thickened filum terminale is frequently present and may be another source of tether. Occasionally dual fila terminales may exist. There is a female predominance in this condition (3.5 F:1 M). Often a cutaneous stigmata, most often hypertrichosis, will suggest the underlying abnormality. Presentation includes the development of an orthopedic deformity, pain, scoliosis, or neurological deficits.

**C. Spinal dermal sinus** is an epithelial-lined tract that can occur at any level of the spine. The importance of these entities is the possibility of communication with the epidural or subdural space and neural elements. They may present with meningitis. Additionally, the tract can cause tethering of the spinal cord and present as such. If the sinus is over the coccyx (below S2) and tracts caudally, it will not communicate with the nervous system.

**D. Neuroectodermal appendages** are tail-like appendages arising in the posterior midline that have sinus tracts extending into the neural canal. It has been proposed that these develop initially as dermal sinus tracts with continued epithelialization outward to form an appendage.

## IV. SACRAL AGENESIS

**A.** Congenital absence of the sacrum in varying degrees occurs in .01–0.5: 1000 live births.

**B. Classification**

1. **Total** sacral agenesis is the complete absence of the sacrum.
2. **Subtotal** sacral agenesis lacks between one and four caudal segments.
3. **Total hemisacrum** agenesis is the complete absence of one half of the sacrum.
4. **Subtotal hemisacrum** agenesis is one or more missing sacral segments in one half of the sacrum.

       **5.Total coccygeal agenesis** is as the name implies.

       **6.Partial coccygeal agenesis** is the partial absence of the coccyx.

  **C. Embryology.** The terms caudal dysplasia, caudal regression, and caudal suppression have been used to describe this condition. The latter term is probably most correct embryologically. The sacrum, which is formed through retrogressive differentiation, can become malformed as a result of embryonic growth constraint.

  **D. Etiology.** Multiple factors have been implicated in the development of sacral agenesis, including embryonic trauma, abnormal osteogenesis of the sacrum during development, maternal diet, and intrapartum pyrexia. Of note, 16% of infants with sacral agenesis have diabetic mothers, suggesting some metabolic contribution.

  **E. Treatment** is primarily preventive and entails the repeated clinical evaluation of affected patients during growth and development. There is a risk of progressive neurological deficits related to a tethered cord.

## V. CRANIORACHISCHISIS

  **A. Encephaloceles** are protrusions of the brain or meninges through a congenital defect in the cranium.

    1.**Incidence** is 1: 5000–10,000 live births, with the highest incidence occurring in Southeast Asia.

    2.In Europe and North America most encephaloceles are located in the posterior cranial vault. In Southeast Asia they are more common in the anterior vault.

    3.Embryologically, these defects are the result of a failure of the anterior neuropore to fuse normally, resulting in various degrees and locations of encephaloceles.

    4.Most encephaloceles are obvious at birth. Encephaloceles of the cranial base may present with nasal obstruction, exophthalmos, or meningitis.

    5.Prognosis is partly based on site, with anterior lesions tending to have a better prognosis than posterior lesions. Associated microcephaly or hydrocephalus are bad prognostic indicators with regard to neurological function.

  **B. Anencephaly (exencephalia acrania)** results when there is failure of the anterior neuropore to close. The brain is absent or very primitive, and there is an associated absence of the cranial vault. Total absence of the spinal cord (amyelia) can be seen in association with anencephaly. There is no treatment for anencephaly and most patients will not survive beyond a few months.

  **C. Dermoid sinuses** at the cranial level are communications between the dermis and the intracranial contents. The communication can be at the level of the bone or the epidural or subdural space, or it may be intraparenchymal. Presentations vary depending on the location and depth of the communication and include meningitis, abscess, hydrocephalus, and mass effect. Treatment is surgical excision of the tract.

  **D. Iniencephaly** is a rare form of craniorachischisis in which the cervical and occipital sclerotomes develop abnormally with resulting defects in the squamous portions of the occipital bone and the cervical vertebrae. The brain herniates through an enlarged foramen magnum.

# Tethered Spinal Cord

An abnormal "tethering" of the spinal cord can result in vascular compromise through mechanical stretching and distortion, causing progressive neurological deficit, orthopedic deformity, and bladder dysfunction. It most commonly occurs as a result of pathology in the lumbosacral region, but can develop in other regions of the spinal canal. This entity is common in a variety of conditions. The diagnosis and management are discussed below.

## I. ASSOCIATED CONDITIONS
   **A.** Myelomeningocele.
   **B.** Lipomyelomeningocele.
   **C.** Lipoma of the filum terminale.
   **D.** Diastematomyelia.
   **E.** Myelocystocele.
   **F.** Neurenteric cyst.
   **G.** Dermoid.
   **H.** Spina bifida occulta.
   **I.** Syringomyelia.
   **J.** Thickened filum terminale.
   **K.** Neuroectodermal appendage.
   **L.** Dermal sinus.
   **M.** Previous surgery.

## II. PATHOPHYSIOLOGY
   **A.** Mechanical distortion of the cord with tethering has been shown experimentally to cause tearing of neuronal membranes.
   **B.** Impaired oxidative metabolism has been demonstrated experimentally in animals with both acute and chronic traction of the spinal cord. Similar studies have been performed on patients undergoing surgical release of a tethered cord. Improved oxidative metabolism after surgical release of the tether has been shown.
   **C.** Blood flow within the tethered spinal cord is impaired locally, causing ischemia of the spinal cord. Blood flow is improved with release.

## III. CLINICAL DIAGNOSIS
   **A. Progressive neurological deficit**
      1. Muscular weakness.
      2. Sensory loss.
      3. Change in bladder function (perhaps the most sensitive indicator).
      4. Change in bowel function.
      5. Change in gait.
      6. Development of, or increase in, spasticity.
   **B. Orthopedic deformity**
      1. Scoliosis.
      2. Kyphosis.
      3. Equinovarus or (rarely) equinovalgus.
      4. Recurrent hip dislocation.
   **C.** Back or leg pain.

**D.** Tenderness on palpation over the tether.
**E. Neurocutaneous stigmata suggesting dysraphism**
1. Capillary hemangioma.
2. Hypertrichosis.
3. Subcutaneous lipoma.
4. Midline color change.
5. Midline dimple.
**F. Acute change after mechanical stress**
1. Lithotomy position.
2. Trauma.
3. Hyperflexion of the spine.
4. Flexion at the hip (e.g., kicking a ball).
**G.** A change in urodynamics, specifically leak pressure measurements and sphincter and detrusor EMG.
**H.** A history of diminished activity or exercise intolerance.

## IV. RADIOGRAPHIC DIAGNOSIS

**A.** MRI can demonstrate a posterior, caudally displaced cord. Scar, lipoma, dermoid, and a tight filum may be seen. If this test is not diagnostic, further studies should be performed. Currently, adjunctive software applications for MRI are being developed with the capacity to detect motion. With further improvements and advances in this technique, MRI may be used as a means to accurately detect cord pulsation.

**B.** Ultrasonography can determine the presence or absence of cord pulsations. A tethered cord will not pulsate normally. This test is only useful in infants and in children with a bony defect overlying the region in question. It is important that the most terminal portions of the cord be visualized, since pulsations can dissipate caudally with tethering.

**C.** Myelogram and postmyelographic CT may define a tether by demonstrating bony, lipomatous, or soft tissue encroachment on the spinal cord. The subarachnoid space will not extend circumferentially around the cord. Again, in cases involving the lumbosacral region, the cord can be displaced posteriorly and caudally (below L2). The filum can be observed to be "tight" and thickened. Dermoids and lipomas may be the source of the tether.

## V. MANAGEMENT is surgical. A laminectomy for the release and resection of the structures (filum terminale, lipoma, dermoid, or scar tissue) causing the tether should be performed.

## VI. INTRAOPERATIVE MANAGEMENT

**A. Magnification** is an essential adjunct to this procedure.

**B. External anal sphincter monitoring** will evaluate changes in the S2–S4 ventral roots.

**C. Electromyography** to assess the remainder of the roots involved. Bilateral hamstring, quadriceps, and anterior tibialis electrodes are commonly placed in addition to the sphincter electrodes. EMG confirmation of level can be particularly useful in cases of myelomeningocele where the anatomy is not normal. Visual observation of the lower extremities during stimulation is very helpful.

**D. Somatosensory evoked potentials** involve stimulation of the common peroneal nerve below the head of the fibula to evaluate conduction times from S1 to the dorsal column. Changes in the latency and amplitude of the SSEP warn that

excessive tension or pressure is being exerted on the conus.
  E. **Pudendal sensory evoked potentials** monitor the S2–S4 dorsal segments through electrodes placed on either side of the penis or between the labia majora and minora. Alteration in the latency or amplification of the waveform suggests excessive pressure on the S2–S4 rootlets.

# VII. POSTOPERATIVE MANAGEMENT
  A. Postoperative pain is optimally managed by an intradural injection of morphine sulfate (0.01 mg/kg) at the time of surgery in patients over 1 year of age. Additional analgesia may not be required for 12–24 hours. The patient should be kept with the head of the bed at a $20^0$ angle to avoid respiratory depression. When necessary, adjunctive intravenous narcotics are effective.
  B. The prone position is most comfortable initially, and this also allows the spinal cord to fall anteriorly (intended to prevent retethering) until the patient is ambulatory.
  C. Early mobilization is preferable. Physical therapy for ambulation should be initiated if the patient does not ambulate well independently. Adequate pain control is helpful in improving mobilization.
  D. Temporary urinary retention can be managed with intermittent catheterization. This will usually return to the preoperative status within 10 days to 3 months. New, permanent urinary dysfunction is an infrequent complication.
  E. Spinal fluid leaks occur infrequently. They can be managed with positioning the head downward, pressure dressings, oversuturing the wound, or continuous subcutaneous catheter drainage if necessary. Surgical re-exploration is rarely required. There is a high incidence of retethering with a postoperative CSF leak.

# VIII. PROGNOSIS
  A. The purpose of operative intervention is to prevent continued neurological deficit and orthopedic deformity. Some improvement in function and scoliosis may occur, in particular in cases with symptoms of a short duration. Surgery is primarily prophylactic. Improvement may not take place, and this point should be made clear to the patient and parent. In most cases, pain will completely resolve.
  B. Retethering remains a risk and at least 10% of patients retether and require re-exploration. The exact incidence of retethering is not known.
  C. Intervention should be sooner rather than later, since the natural history of the disease is a progressive decline in function.

# Hydrocephalus

Hydrocephalus is a pathological condition with a multitude of etiologies. It is a condition that results from an imbalance in CSF production and absorption such that more CSF is produced than is absorbed. This condition can be the result of an obstructive process within the ventricle or subarachnoid space. Rarely, it can result from an increase in CSF production, such as may occur with a choroid plexus papilloma. The classification, etiology, diagnosis, and treatment are discussed below.

## I. GENERAL
   A. The reported incidence of congenital hydrocephalus is 3–4 : 1000 live births.
   B. As a single congenital disorder, hydrocephalus occurs in 0.9–1.5 : 1000 live births.
   C. In association with spina bifida, hydrocephalus occurs in 1.3–2.9 : 1000 live births; 95% of children with spina bifida will develop hydrocephalus.
   D. In general, hydrocephalics produce less CSF than normal individuals.
   E. It has also been noted that the metabolism of the surrounding brain is diminished in hydrocephalus.

## II. CLASSIFICATION AND ETIOLOGY
   A. Historically hydrocephalus has been described as communicating or noncommunicating. These terms were initiated to describe the impact of the pathological condition on CSF circulation. This differentiation is important with regard to treatment. For example, if communicating hydrocephalus is present, third ventriculoscopy is not a useful treatment, and if noncommunicating hydrocephalus is present, a lumboperitoneal shunt will not be effective. The terms obstructive and nonobstructive may be more appropriate, although almost all cases of hydrocephalus have some element of obstruction to CSF absorption.
   B. **Noncommunicating hydrocephalus** is produced by a process which obstructs the ventricular system.
      1. **Acquired**
         a. **Tumors,** most commonly fourth ventricular tumors such as medulloblastoma or ependymoma, although other tumors may cause hydrocephalus as well.
         b. **Fibrosis of the leptomeninges** as a result of meningitis or intraventricular hemorrhage.
         c. **Aqueductal stenosis** is usually secondary to gliosis. Tectal gliomas may present as late-onset aqueductal stenosis. With aqueductal stenosis the lateral and third ventricles are enlarged and the fourth is normal in size.
      2. **Congenital**
         a. **Aqueductal stenosis** occurs in a variety of forms. Aqueductal *forking* may be seen in association with myelomeningocele and ACM. A septum, or true narrowing, may be present, causing the stenosis. Characteristi-

cally, the posterior fossa is small in cases of congenital
aqueductal stenosis.

   **b. Dandy-Walker syndrome** is characterized by a cystic
dilatation of the fourth ventricle with absent or hypoplastic cerebellum and elevation of the torcula. Atresia of the
foramina of Magendie and Luschka during embryogenesis may play a role in its development.

   **c. Vein of Galen aneurysms** and other vascular malformations can cause hydrocephalus.

   **d. Benign intracranial cysts** such as arachnoid cysts and
ependymal cysts.

   **e. Tumors.**

   **f. X-linked hydrocephalus** accounts for rare cases of
congenital hydrocephalus in males.

**C. Communicating hydrocephalus** occurs when there is an
obstruction to CSF flow distal to the outlets of the fourth
ventricle or at the level of the pacchionian granulations.

  **1. Acquired**

    **a. Leptomeningeal inflammation** can develop secondary to meningitis or intraventricular hemorrhage.

    **b. Venous thrombosis** can cause hydrocephalus. Partial
venous sinus stenosis may explain why patients continue
with hydrocephalus after the resection of a posterior
fossa tumor.

    **c. Carcinomatous meningitis** can result from neoplastic
involvement of the basal cisterns.

    **d. Trauma** resulting in subarachnoid blood with subsequent inflammatory reaction in the arachnoid can result
in acquired hydrocephalus.

  **2. Congenital**

    **a. Leptomeningeal inflammation.**

    **b. Encephaloceles.**

    **c. Lissencephaly (agyria).**

    **d. Platybasia (basilar invagination).**

**D. Functional hydrocephalus** can develop as a result of
oversecretion of CSF by a choroid plexus papilloma. The
tumor itself may obstruct the ventricular system and result
in noncommunicating hydrocephalus. In other cases, small
hemorrhages from these tumors may cause obstruction of the
subarachnoid pathways. The latter is the explanation for the
persistence of hydrocephalus that is seen in some cases after
tumor removal.

**E. Hydrocephalus ex vacuo** is enlargement of the ventricular system secondary to atrophy. This is not true
hydrocephalus because CSF production equals absorption.
Radiographic workup demonstrates an increase in ventricular size with signs of atrophy (i.e., generous sulci). The head
will be small to normal in size (depending on the age at the
time of the insult) and grow at a decelerated rate.

**F. Normal pressure hydrocephalus** is usually seen in adults
and is not a pediatric disease. It refers to hydrocephalus
associated with a physiological CSF pressure. This condition
exists when there is an incomplete block of the CSF pathways, allowing for equilibration of CSF pressures to a physiologic range. Over time, stretching of the neuronal fibers may

lead to progressive white matter wasting. The classical clinical triad is dementia, ataxia, and urinary incontinence.

## III. HYDROCEPHALUS AND PREMATURITY

A. Yearly, over 35,000 infants weighing less than 1 kg are born in the United States. Among infants weighing less than 1500 g, 35–70% will develop IVH; 20–50% of these will go on to develop ventriculomegaly.

B. The immature germinal matrix is the source of hemorrhage.

C. Hemorrhage usually occurs within 48 hours of birth, with 50% of cases occurring within the first 24 hours.

D. Surveillance with the daily measurement of head circumference, serial cranial ultrasound, and examination of the fontanelle and sutures enables the diagnosis of IVH and monitors for the development of hydrocephalus.

E. Treatment with lumbar punctures is recommended initially. If these are technically not feasible, or inadequate, then a subcutaneous ventricular reservoir (or some type of CSF drainage system) for daily CSF withdrawal is recommended.

F. Shunting should be performed when the infant has grown, is medically stable, and CSF protein is decreased.

## IV. CLINICAL DIAGNOSIS

A. At birth, congenital hydrocephalus may be grossly apparent by the following features:
  1. Abnormally large head.
  2. Thin skin.
  3. Paresis of upgaze—"sunsetting."
  4. Transillumination of the skull.
  5. Bulging scalp veins.
  6. Split sutures.
  7. Bulging fontanelle.

B. Postnatal diagnosis has the following salient features:
  1. Excessive rate of head growth (growth which crosses percentile lines).
  2. Bulging or tense anterior fontanelle with loss of pulsations.
  3. Loss of, or failure to achieve, developmental milestones.
  4. Irritability.
  5. Poor feeding.
  6. "Cracked pot" sound on percussing the skull.
  7. Split sutures.
  8. "Sunsetting."
  9. Papilledema.

C. **Hereditary macrocrania** should be distinguished from hydrocephalus. It is characterized by a normal rate of head growth and a familial occurrence of macrocrania.

## V. RADIOGRAPHIC DIAGNOSIS

A. **Plain x-ray** may reveal a "beaten metal" appearance of the skull and split sutures. X-rays may suggest the type of hydrocephalus, i.e., a small posterior fossa suggests aqueductal stenosis and a large posterior fossa a Dandy-Walker syndrome.

B. **Ultrasound** assesses the degree of ventricular enlargement and may reveal intraventricular hemorrhage. It is an easy, inexpensive bedside test particularly well suited to the medically labile premature infant. It can be used for follow-up examinations as long as the fontanelle remains open. This modality is also useful for intrauterine diagnosis of hydrocephalus.

C. **CT scan** defines the ventricular system with greater accuracy and reveals septations which may be present within the ventricular system. It will also disclose underlying abnormalities such as ACM. In the case of obstructive hydrocephalus related to tumor or vascular anomalies, this study is particularly useful. With loculated ventricular systems, the injection of a contrast medium into various chambers is useful to determine communications.

D. **MRI** should be reserved for hydrocephalus associated with tumors or vascular malformations, and loculated or septated ventricular systems.

E. **Angiogram** is indicated in cases of hydrocephalus associated with vein of Galen malformations and other vascular anomalies.

## VI. TREATMENT

A. Removing the obstruction to CSF absorption when feasible (i.e., tumor).

B. Shunting CSF to a body cavity where it will be absorbed.

C. Commonly utilized shunt systems include ventriculoperitoneal, ventriculoatrial, and lumboperitoneal shunts. Ventriculopleural shunts and ventriculocisternostomy (Torkildsen's) are used less commonly. Ventriculogallbladder and ventriculoureteral shunts are rarely used.

D. **Third ventriculostomy** is the surgical creation of a connection between the third ventricle and the interpeduncular cistern.

E. There are no medications which will adequately treat hydrocephalus. However, acetazolamide or furosemide may be a useful adjunct in some patients.

## VII. FOLLOW-UP

A. Children with shunts need to be followed by a neurosurgeon for life.

B. Infants should be followed with greater frequency because of the risk of insidious shunt malfunction.

C. Initially and immediately after shunt revisions, children should be seen more frequently, with the frequency of exams being spaced to yearly intervals gradually after birth or revision.

# Shunt Equipment

Hydrocephalus is managed by the diversion of CSF to a body cavity which has the capacity to absorb spinal fluid. A variety of shunt apparatus is available. The myriad of equipment produced suggests that the ideal system does not exist. Preference of shunt apparatus is unique to each neurosurgeon. A variety of systems are described.

I. **TYPES OF SHUNTS.** The ventriculoperitoneal shunt is the most commonly used shunt apparatus; however, a variety of shunts have been devised and are listed below.
   A. Ventriculoperitoneal.
   B. Ventriculoatrial.
   C. Ventriculopleural.
   D. Lumboperitoneal.
   E. Torkildsen's (ventriculocisternostomy).
   F. Ventriculogallbladder.
   G. Others of historical interest
      1. Fallopian tube.
      2. Mastoid process.
      3. Ureter.
      4. Thoracic duct.
      5. Salivary duct.
      6. Stomach/ileum.
      7. Spinal epidural space.
      8. Subdural space.
      9. Sagittal sinus.
II. **COMPONENTS.** Many types of shunt equipment by various manufacturers are available. Not all are listed below, but the basic types are reviewed. Regardless of the type of shunt, most shunts have three major components. The components may be one integral unit or connected by connectors. With the exception of the valve and connectors, most components are radiopaque to allow for x-ray examination.
   A. **Intraventricular catheter**
      1. Classical placement is with the distal tip in the lateral ventricle, anterior to the foramen of Monro to minimize contact with the choroid plexus. Isolated ventricles may necessitate alternate placement as needed.
      2. **Phlanged catheters,** once thought to prevent proximal obstruction, are seldom used today. Their removal can be hazardous.
   B. **Shunt devices**
      1. **Valves**
         a. Provide unidirectional flow.
         b. Avoid reflux.
         c. Variable opening pressures: low (5–50 mm $H_2O$); medium (51–110 mm $H_2O$); high (111–180 mm $H_2O$), or variable resistance valves, which diminish siphoning.
      2. Types of shunt devices
         a. **Unishunt.** An integral shunt unit as opposed to one

composed of pieces connected at the time of placement.
  b. **Double-dome reservoir.** Pressure over the proximal dome while pumping the distal dome evaluates distal patency. The reverse assesses proximal function.
  c. **Multipurpose valves** are composed of (from proximal to distal) a proximal occluder, a dome reservoir, and an on-off switch that can be followed by an antisiphon device. The switch is turned off by percutaneously manipulating a Silastic ball into a cup to prevent distal flow. Flow is re-established by putting pressure on the proximal occluder and pumping the dome reservoir to release the ball.
  d. **Antisiphon devices** close when there is negative pressure distally. They may be mistaken for reservoirs. Care should be taken not to tap this device as it can be damaged.
  e. **Burr hole valves** have a dome that serves as a valve, pump, and reservoir. These may be difficult to palpate as they are seated within a burr hole.
  f. **Holter valve systems** are cylindrical devices with unidirectional stainless steel valves proximally and a distal silicone pumping chamber that can be damaged with tapping. A proximal reservoir may be present to allow for CSF access.
  g. **Hakim shunts** are composed of a proximal reservoir with a metal base for sampling of CSF, and a cylindrical valve system with stainless steel valves surrounding a silicone pumping chamber.
  h. The **Denver shunt** is a flow-regulated shunt rather than a pressure-regulated system. It has a Silastic pumping chamber with a proximal slit valve and a distal catheter with slit valves. A tapping reservoir may be inserted proximally.
  i. **Variable resistance** valves such as the Delta and Omega-Sigma valves are now available.
  j. **Programmable shunts** for both variable resistance and pressure are currently being developed.
C. **Distal catheter**
  1. Tubing with distal perforations.
  2. Open Silastic tube.
  3. Distal slit valve.
  4. Raimondi tubing has wire coils to prevent kinking. These are more commonly associated with bowel perforations than Silastic tubing.

# Shunt Infection

Shunt infection is the most significant of all shunt complications. It is the cause of significant morbidity and even mortality. This chapter deals with the prevention, diagnosis, and management of shunt infections.

## I. INCIDENCE

A. The incidence of shunt infection is from 2–38%. This varies tremendously from institution to institution and between surgeons. An acceptable range is probably less than 5%.

B. The surgeon is the largest single factor affecting the incidence of shunt infection.

C. Factors associated with higher infection rates.

1. Successive shunt revisions.
2. Shunts in children with myelomeningocele.
3. Children less than 6 months of age.
4. Premature infants.

## II. PREVENTION

A. **Operative technique.** Attention to meticulous technique from the skin preparation to the application of the dressing provides the best prevention from infection. Shorter operative times are associated with lower infection rates.

B. **Adjunctive equipment.** Surgical isolation bubbles are an effective adjunct against infection. While still early in development, Silastic impregnated with antimicrobials is a promising adjunct.

C. **Prophylactic antibiotics.** While prospective, randomized studies have not found a statistical difference in infection rate with prophylactic antibiotics, most centers continue to use them. Prophylactic agents are selected to prevent *Staphylococcus epidermidis* infections. The agents should be selected based on hospital infection patterns. Therapy should be initiated approximately 1 hour prior to surgery. Table 12-1 lists dosages of the most commonly used agents.

## III. CLINICAL PRESENTATION

A. History of a recent shunt operation or surgical procedure involving the body cavity in which the shunt catheter resides. Seventy percent of infections are apparent within 2 months of surgery. Greater than 80% are manifested within 6 months. Infections which present in the first 2 to 3 days are most commonly gram-negative infections. Cases presenting in the first few weeks to months are likely to be staphylococcus and diphtheroid infections.

B. Signs and symptoms of shunt malfunction

1. Fever.
2. Irritability.
3. Change in sensorium.
4. Swelling or erythema around the shunt tube.
5. Ventriculoatrial shunts may present with sepsis, shunt nephritis, or signs of septic emboli.

## IV. DIAGNOSIS

A. Clinical presentation (see sec. III).

**Table 12-1. Prophylactic antibiotics (neonates > 2 kg)**

| Agent | Dosage (mg/kg) |
| --- | --- |
| **Intravenous** | |
| Nafcillin | Neonates 0–6 days 50–100/24h div q12h<br>Neonates 7–28 days 100–200/24h div q6–8h<br>Children 50–200/24h div q6h |
| Vancomycin | Neonates 0–7 days 10 q12h<br>Neonates >7 days 10 q8h<br>Older infants and children 30–45/24h div q8 |
| Ceftriaxone | Neonates 50–75/24h div q12–24h (max 2 gms/day)<br>Children 50–75/24h div q12h |
| Cefotaxime | Neonates 0–7 days 50 q12h<br>Neonates 8–28 days 50 q8h<br>Children 50–180/24h div q4–6h (max 12 gms/day) |
| Oxacillin | Neonates 0–7 days 25 q8h<br>Neonates >7 days 25 q6h<br>Children 75/24h div q6h |
| Gentamycin | Neonates 1–7 days 2.5 q12h<br>Neonates >7 days and infants 2.5 q8h<br>Children 2–2.5 q8h |
| Methicillin | Neonates 0–7 days 25 q8h<br>Neonates 8–28 days 25 q6h<br>Children 100–400/24h div q4–6h |
| **Oral** | |
| Co-trimoxazole | Children 4 mg/kg trimethoprim per 20mg/kg sulfamethoxazole q12h |

B. Examination of CSF from a shunt tap demonstrates an elevated leukocyte count with increased segmented cells, elevated protein levels, diminished glucose levels, and ultimately a positive culture. Lumbar puncture may be negative in the setting of a shunt infection and should not be used as a means of ruling out shunt infection.

C. Gram's stain is positive in a majority of *Staphylococcus* and gram-negative bacillary infections.

D. Shunt taps provide CSF for examination as well as provide information about shunt function, i.e., the ability to aspirate fluid.

E. Occult infections with indolent bacteria *(Propionibacterium)* are being recognized more frequently. Cultures should be maintained for 10 to 14 days to ensure the diagnosis of infections with these indolent bacteria and anaerobic infections.

## V. MICROBIOLOGY

A. *S. epidermidis* is the leading cause of shunt infections. *Staphylococcus aureus* accounts for 25% of all shunt infections.

B. Gram-negative enteric bacteria (*Klebsiella, Escherichia coli, Proteus*) cause a number of infections. The remainder of infections are caused by *Haemophilus influenzae, Streptococcus pneumoniae,* and *Neisseria meningitidis.* Delayed infections are frequently due to *Propionibacterium.*

## VI. PATHOGENESIS

A. Direct inoculation at surgery.

B. Retrograde travel from a contaminated distal catheter.

C. Hematogenous spread (rare except with ventriculoatrial shunts).

## VII. MANAGEMENT

A. In patients who present with shunt malfunction and shunt infection, the shunt should be removed and external ventricular drainage instituted. Intravenous antibiotics with or without intraventricular antibiotics, depending on CSF penetration and sensitivities, should be administered until CSF sterility is achieved. A new shunt system is then inserted.

B. In patients without shunt malfunction, the shunt can be left in place and intravenous (with or without intrashunt) antibiotics are administered until CSF sterility is achieved. The shunt is then removed, and a new system inserted. Intravenous antibiotics are then continued for 7 days. This alternative is associated with the highest cure rate. Attempts made to sterilize the shunt in situ without replacement are less effective.

C. The selection of antibiotics for intraventricular or intrashunt and intravenous use should be broad-spectrum or based on Gram's stain of the CSF. These agents can be changed as cultures and sensitivities become available (Table 12-2). Table 12-3 gives dosages for commonly used agents in the management of shunt infections.

D. *H. influenzae* meningitis in a child with a shunt can be successfully treated without shunt removal.

## VIII. PROGNOSIS

A. Children with a history of shunt infection have lower IQs (73 +/-26 SD) than those who have not suffered an infection (95 +/- 19 SD).

B. The severity of the infection has not been correlated with the degree of intellectual decline. There is, however, a trend for gram-negative infections to cause a greater decline in IQ.

C. The mortality associated with shunt infection was 5–10% in 1976. Since then, it has declined further, and is now minimal.

**Table 12-2. Intrashunt and intravenous antibiotic selection based on organism**

| Organism | Intrashunt | Intravenous |
|---|---|---|
| *S. epidermidis* <br> *S. aureus* | Vancomycin | Vancomycin <br> Rifampin and TMP-SMZ |
| Enterococcus | Vancomycin <br> Gentamycin | Vancomycin |
| Other Streptococci <br>   PCN m.i.c. < = 0.1 | Gentamycin | Penicillin G |
|   PCN m.i.c. > = 0.2 | Vancomycin <br> Gentamycin | Penicillin G |
| Aerobic gram-negative rods | Gentamycin | Cefotaxime |
| Diphtheroids | Vancomycin | Vancomycin <br> TMP-SMZ |

PCN= penicillin; TMP-SMZ = co-trimoxazole; m.i.c.= minimum inhibitory concentration.

**Table 12-3. Antibiotics used in the treatment of shunt infection (neonates > 2 kg)**

| Agent | Dosage (mg/kg) |
|---|---|
| **Intravenous** | |
| Vancomycin | Neonates 0–7 days 10 q12h <br> Neonates >7 days 10 q8h <br> Older infants and children 30–45/24h div q8h |
| Gentamycin | Neonates 1–7 days 2.5 q12h <br> Neonates >7 days and infants 2.5 q8h <br> Children 2–2.5 q8h |
| Nafcillin | Neonates 0–6 days 50–100/24h div q12h <br> Neonates 7–28 days 100–200/24h div q6-8h <br> Children 100–200/24h div q4–6h |
| Cefotaxime | Neonates 0–7 days 50 q12h <br> Neonates 8–28 days 50 q8h <br> Children 50–180/24h div q4–6h (max 12 gms/day) |
| Ceftazidime | Neonates < 28 days 30 q12h <br> Infants and children 30–50 q8h |

**Table 12-3.** *(continued)*

| Agent | Dosage (mg/kg) |
|---|---|
| Ceftriaxone | Neonates 50–75/24h div q12–24h (max 2 gms/day)<br>Children 50–75/24h div q12h |
| Penicillin G | Neonates < 7 days 100,000–150,000 U/kg/24h<br>  div q8h<br>Neonates 7–28 days 200,000 U/kg/24h div q6h<br>Infants and children 100,000–400,000 U/kg/24h<br>  div q4–6h |

**Oral**

| | |
|---|---|
| Rifampin | Children >5 years 10–20 q24h single dose<br>  (max 600 mg/24h) |
| Co-trimoxazole | Children 4 mg/kg trimethoprim per 20<br>  mg/kg sulfamethoxazole q12h |

**Intrashunt**

| | |
|---|---|
| Vancomycin | 5–10 mg qd (trough CSF level 10 mcg/ml) |
| Gentamycin | 8 mg qd (trough CSF level 4 mcg/ml) |

# Shunt Complications

Shunt procedures are accompanied by a variety of shunt complications. Infection is the most significant shunt complication and is dealt with in Chapter 12. Because of mechanical failure, the majority of shunt patients will require revision by the time the shunt has been in place for 10 years. This chapter addresses these types of complications as well as the surgical complications of shunting.

**I. MECHANICAL FAILURE** represents the leading cause of shunt malfunction.

    **A. Obstruction** may occur related to plugging of the ventricular catheter with choroid plexus, brain, or protein. The latter occurs at the distal end as well. Shunts placed in conjunction with tumors may become obstructed by tumor cells. Premature infants shunted for IVH have a higher level of protein for several months and are predisposed to obstruction. Whenever a protein plug is present, infection must be ruled out.

    **B. Disconnection** can occur at any point in the system. Obviously, sites of connection and mobility are at risk. Shunts that have been in place for some time may break as they become fixed and the patient grows. The continuity of a shunt can be assessed by palpation, but the fibrous tract may feel and even act like tubing. A CSF collection may be present over a shunt disconnection. X-ray examination (AP/lateral skull, chest, and KUB) is definitive. Note that some portions of the shunt system, such as the valve and connectors can be radiolucent and appear to represent disconnections.

    **C. Migration** may result in shunt malfunction. With growth, the distal end of a vascular shunt can leave the atrium and become dysfunctional. Shunts can migrate into the scrotum or a loculation within the peritoneal cavity, thereby compromising function. Migration to a variety of sites has been reported, including the chest, umbilicus, rectum, vagina, intrahepatic, and intracranial.

**II. DISTAL CATHETER** problems occur in a variety of settings.

    **A. Abdominal procedures** for appendicitis or urological procedures may cause subsequent shunt malfunction due to infection or poor peritoneal absorption.

    **B. Pseudocyst** formation may impair CSF absorption. Smaller cysts tend to be related to infection, while larger cysts are often sterile.

    **C. Preperitoneal placement** may present with sudden shunt malfunction.

    **D. Migration** (see sec. I. C.)

**III. PROXIMAL CATHETER**

    **A. Hemorrhage** at the time of placement is unusual. In catheters that are removed after being in situ for some time, there is an increased risk of hemorrhage intraoperatively. If this occurs, the intraventricular blood may cause subsequent obstruction.

    **B. Pneumocephalus** may be present, in particular in shunts placed in association with tumor resection. This can cause an "air lock" and subsequent shunt malfunction. Shunt pumping for several days may help clear air from the system.

**C. Seizures** occur at a rate of 5–48% in children with shunts. Shunt infection and malfunction should be ruled out if new seizures occur. Once this has been assessed, they should be managed with appropriate anticonvulsant therapy.

**D. Short catheters** placed in cases of massive hydrocephalus will malfunction as the cerebral mantle expands. Adequate catheter length is essential at initial operation.

**IV. VALVES** come in a variety of opening pressures. They do not usually fail in and of themselves, but may cause shunt malfunction if an inappropriate pressure has been selected for a patient. A valve with too high an opening pressure will not relieve the symptoms of increased intracranial pressure. A valve with too low an opening pressure may cause the development of subdural hematomas with overdrainage. A variety of mechanical devices are available to prevent overdrainage.

**V. VENTRICULAR ANOMALIES** can contribute to shunt malfunction.

**A. Loculated ventricles** often develop as a result of infection. Other causes include Dandy-Walker syndrome and severe IVH. Assessment of communication can be readily performed with intraventricular injections of contrast material followed by delayed CT scanning. All symptomatic, isolated CSF collections which cause mass effect must be drained with separate catheters or communicated to the shunt with craniotomy or ventriculoscopy. Loculations in an otherwise routine case of hydrocephalus should raise concern for the possibility of infection.

**B. Slit ventricle syndrome** is the association of episodic signs and symptoms of increased intracranial pressure in patients with small or slit-like ventricular systems. This is an uncommon syndrome. Treatment options include furosemide, acetazolamide, steroids, shunt revision, and craniectomy. A variety of mechanisms have been proposed to explain this syndrome:

1. Overdrainage of CSF.
2. Intermittent shunt malfunction with mild increases in ventricular size causing symptoms.
3. Periventricular fibrosis.
4. Decreased intracranial compliance.

**VI. VASCULAR SHUNTS** are associated with some unique complications such as shunt nephritis, pulmonary embolism, cor pulmonale, and sepsis.

**VII. SURGICAL**

**A. Retained fragments** usually occur with revisions of systems that have been in place for some time. Catheters may adhere to the choroid plexus, making removal both difficult and dangerous. In these cases, it is usually preferable to leave the catheter behind. Fragments may fracture within the tract from the head to the abdomen. When there is no foreign body reaction these may be left behind. Peritoneal catheters that have become disconnected and are not easily accessible may also be left behind. These fragments are usually harmless, except in cases where infection develops, in which case their removal is a prerequisite to clear the infection.

B. **Bowel perforation** may occur with peritoneal catheter placement. Patients with prior abdominal procedures should undergo distal catheter placement under direct vision. An increase in bowel perforation using the peritoneal trocar is **not** noted in properly selected patients.

C. **Bladder perforation** may occur in patients who have undergone bladder augmentations (in particular those with neurogenic bladders). Again, in these cases placement into the peritoneum should be under direct vision.

# Phakomatoses

The neurocutaneous disorders (phakomatoses) are a group of disorders characterized by neurological, ocular, and cutaneous involvement. These are genetic disorders with a natural history of progressive involvement with age. Early recognition of a phakomatosis allows for genetic counseling of the patient, siblings, and offspring, as well as providing optimal medical surveillance and care. The precise genes for a number of these disorders are currently being discovered.

## I. NEUROFIBROMATOSIS
### A. General
1. NF is the most common phakomatosis, with an incidence of 1:3000 live births.
2. Autosomal dominant disorder with variable clinical expression. Penetrance approaches 100%. Fifty percent of new cases occur as mutations.
3. NF appears in two distinct forms, **peripheral NF** (classic von Recklinghausen's NF) and **central NF** (bilateral acoustic NF).
4. Hallmarks of the disease include multiple pigmented spots on the skin (café au lait spots) and multiple neurofibromas.

### B. Peripheral NF
1. Features
   a. **Cutaneous neurofibromas** vary in number and size. Neurofibromas develop on peripheral nerves, nerve roots, and the sympathetic chain. Pathologically they consist of Schwann cells, fibroblasts, mast cells, and connective tissue.
   b. **Café au lait spots** are hyperpigmented spots usually visible over the trunk.
   c. **Pigmented iris hamartomas** (Lisch nodules) are present in the majority of patients over 6 years of age and increase in number with age.
   d. **Freckles** involving intertriginous areas (axilla, buttocks).
   e. **Plexiform neurofibromas** may be associated with peripheral nerves of the sympathetic chain. They may grow considerably and result in hemihypertrophy (elephantiasis neuromatosa). They can also undergo sarcomatous degeneration into neurofibrosarcoma as suggested by rapid enlargement.
   f. **Buphthalmos** (ox eye) results from glaucoma causing an enlargement of the globe. It is most commonly unilateral.
   g. **Scoliosis** is the most common skeletal malformation associated with NF. Surgical intervention can help prevent severe deformity.
2. **Diagnosis.** The diagnosis is based on clinical criteria and family history. In pediatric patients, five spots larger than 5 mm in diameter suggest a diagnosis of PNF. These are

optimally counted using a Wood's lamp. However, 20% of patients with PNF do not fulfill this criteria, so this is not absolute. The presence of neurofibromas and/or Lisch nodules contributes to the diagnosis. A family history of NF is useful, but not essential, as it can occur as a new mutation.

**3. Treatment** is expectant. Symptomatic neurofibromas can be surgically excised, although with some risk to function. Genetic counseling is an essential part of therapy.

**4. Prognosis.** PNF is a progressive disorder. Prognosis depends on the degree of expression. The tendency is toward progressive problems. If sarcomatous changes occur in a neurofibroma, there is only a 23% 5-year survival rate.

## C. Central NF
### 1. Features
  **a.** Bilateral acoustic neuromas usually becoming symptomatic in adolescence.
  **b.** Cutaneous neurofibromas (less than in PNF).
  **c.** Café au lait spots (less than PNF).
  **d.** Congenital cataracts.
### 2. Diagnosis
  **a.** CT or MRI of the brain.
  **b.** BAER may detect small acoustic neuromas.
  **c.** Family history
### 3. Treatment is again expectant. With MRI, acoustic tumors can be diagnosed when very small. Currently, a tendency toward earlier operation is developing. The results from these patients over the next several decades will decide the benefits of this course of management. Genetic counseling is an essential part of therapy.
### 4. Prognosis. CNF is a progressive disorder. Removal of acoustic tumors while sparing hearing and facial function is of paramount concern. Sarcomatous degeneration of tumors carries a poor prognosis.

## D. CNS involvement (PNF and CNF)
  **1.** Lesions of the brain, cranial nerves, spinal cord, nerve roots, and meninges develop in PNF and CNF.
  **2.** In general, lesions need to be managed surgically when symptomatic. Asymptomatic lesions need to be assessed and managed on a case-by-case basis. Frequently multiple tumors prevent the excision of all lesions.
  **3.** Optic gliomas are common in children with NF. This tumor has a better prognosis in the setting of NF than in other "normal" children. This may be the initial presentation of NF in children.
  **4.** Gliomas also occur in other regions of the CNS. Hypothalamic involvement is suggested by precocious puberty or sexual infantilism.
  **5.** Meningiomas (intracranial or spinal).
  **6.** Spinal neurofibromas are common.
  **7. Sequelae**
    **a.** Seizures.
    **b.** Macrocephaly (75%).
    **c.** Developmental delay.
    **d.** Learning disabilities.

      **e.** Mental retardation.
- **E. Segmental neurofibromatosis.** The presence of café au lait spots and neurofibromatoses within a limited area of the upper body (i.e., half the trunk and an arm).
- **F. Cutaneous neurofibromatosis.** The presence of café au lait spots only.

## II. TUBEROUS SCLEROSIS

### A. General
1. Autosomal dominant inheritance with a large number of sporadic cases.
2. **Incidence** of 1:10,000 live births. It is more common in males and uncommon in blacks.
3. TS involves the central nervous system, skin, viscera, retina, kidneys, and bone.
4. The classic triad consists of adenoma sebaceum, mental retardation, and seizures.
5. **Bourneville's disease.** TS with involvement of the CNS.
6. **Pringle's disease.** TS with only cutaneous lesions.
7. **West syndrome.** Cutaneous lesions associated with mental retardation, infantile spasms, and hypsarrhythmia.

### B. Features
1. **Ash leaf spots** are depigmented skin spots which are pointed at one end, and rounded on the other. They may be present at birth or appear later in childhood. A Wood's lamp may help visualize these spots, particularly in the fair-skinned.
2. **Adenoma sebaceum** (facial angiofibromas) are reddened, raised hamartomas arising from nervous elements of the skin. They are present in 90% of TS patients.
3. **Subungual angiofibromas** on the fingers and toes.
4. **Subependymal fibrosis** (sharkskin).
5. **Retinal lesions** comprised of glia, ganglion cells, and fibroblasts.
6. Renal hamartomas, angiomyolipomas, and cysts.
7. Cardiac rhabdomyomas.
8. Hepatic hamartomas and angiomas.
9. Pulmonary lymphangiomatosis.
10. Skeletal abnormalities (cystic defects, osteosclerosis).

### C. CNS involvement
1. **Subependymal nodules** project into the third and lateral ventricles and may be partially embedded in the thalamus or caudate nucleus. Histologically, these are composed of elongated, gemistocytic astrocytes with frequent calcification.
2. **Cortical nodules** ("tubers") occur primarily in the cerebral cortex. Pathologically they appear to be areas of focally enlarged cortical tissue with abnormal neurons, astrocytes, and cytoarchitecture.
3. **Subependymal giant cell astrocytomas** arise in 7–23% of patients with TS. They commonly occur at the foramen of Monro and present with signs of increased ICP from obstructive hydrocephalus.
4. Pachygyria, microgyria, and various heterotopias.
5. Vascular hyperplasia.

**D. Diagnosis.** Patients usually come to medical attention with a seizure disorder. CT or MRI scan shows the pathognomonic lesions. Full workup discloses some of the other manifestations. Rarely, patients come to medical attention with renal symptoms (azotemia, hypertension, albuminuria).

**E. Treatment**
1. Seizure control.
2. Neurosurgical intervention for tumors causing intractable seizures, or hydrocephalus.
3. Laser therapy or dermabrasion of facial lesions.
4. Genetic counseling.

**F. Prognosis.** Seizures prior to the age of 2 portend a grave prognosis and these patients are likely to be severely mentally retarded. Patients without seizures may have normal mentation.

## III. VON HIPPEL-LINDAU DISEASE (retinocerebellar angiomatosis)

**A. General**
1. This is an autosomal dominant disorder with variable expression that usually presents in adults.
2. Solitary hemangioblastomas may be seen in children without VL.

**B. Features**
1. **Capillary hemangioblastomas** (tumors composed of embryonic vascular elements) are the most common lesions of VL. The most common location for these is the cerebellum but they do occur throughout the craniospinal axis.
2. Retinal angiomas.
3. Pheochromocytoma.
4. Renal cysts, tumors, and angiomas.
5. Angiomas of the pancreas, liver, spleen, lung, epididymis.

**C. Diagnosis.** The diagnosis of VL is reserved for those patients with more than one separate lesion or a single lesion and a positive family history.

**D. Treatment** of symptomatic hemangioblastomas is surgical. Spinal hemangioblastomas may be associated with syringomyelia.

**E. Prognosis.** VL is a progressive disorder. Periodic radiographic screening and renal studies with surgical management of symptomatic lesions is recommended. Genetic counseling is imperative.

## IV. NEUROCUTANEOUS ANGIOMATOSES

**A. Sturge-Weber syndrome** (encephalotrigeminal angiomatosis)
1. Sporadic incidence suggesting mutation.
2. **Features.** Port-wine nevus of the face in the first or second division of the trigeminal nerve with ipsilateral leptomeningeal angiomatosis, usually parietal and occipital. Cortical atrophy and calcification can develop below the meningeal abnormality. In some cases angiomas arise in other parts of the body.
3. **Clinical presentation.** Seizures, contralateral hemiparesis, ipsilateral glaucoma, homonymous hemianopsia, and, in more severe cases, mental retarda-

tion.
4. **Radiographic studies.** Plain x-rays show "trolley-track" calcifications along the cerebral convolutions. CT demonstrates intracranial calcifications, meningeal angiomatous malformation, and unilateral cerebral atrophy.
5. **Treatment** is aimed at seizure control. Surgery (hemispherectomy, lobectomy) needs to be considered, especially with the early onset of seizures.
6. **Prognosis** varies from patient to patient. Extensive cerebral involvement and early onset of seizures suggest a poor prognosis. Patients with normal intelligence, good seizure control, and only mild hemiparesis have been described.

B. **Osler-Rendu-Weber** syndrome
1. Autosomal dominant inheritance.
2. **Features.** Angiomas of the skin, mucous membranes, and nervous system.
3. Angiomas within the central nervous system may hemorrhage or become otherwise symptomatic, requiring neurosurgical intervention.

C. **Fabry's disease** (angiokeratoma corporis diffusum)
1. X-linked disorder causing a defect of alpha-galactosidase A, with an accumulation of trihexosyl-ceramide in a variety of cells and tissues.
2. **Features.** Corneal opacities and multiple purple macular and maculopapular hyperkeratotic lesions over the abdomen and lower extremities.
3. **Clinical presentation.** Pain and burning in the limbs, anhydrosis, and renal failure.
4. **Treatment.** Phenytoin has been reported to improve pain symptoms. Renal transplant should be considered with the onset of renal failure.
5. **Prognosis.** The disease is progressive. Cerebrovascular accidents, renal failure, and myocardial involvement may occur.

D. **Ataxia-telangiectasia** (Louis-Bar syndrome)
1. Autosomal recessive transmission with an incidence of 2–3: 100,000 live births.
2. **Features.** Progressive ataxia, multiple telangiectasias, immunodeficiency, and an increased incidence of neoplasia.
3. **Clinical presentation.** The development of progressive ataxia, dysarthria, and choreoathetosis during childhood.
4. **Radiographic studies** show cerebellar atrophy most prominent in the vermis, and demyelination evident in the brainstem and spinal cord.
5. **Treatment** involves management of infections due to immunologic deficiencies, physical therapy, and other supportive care.
6. The **prognosis** is poor, with most patients requiring wheelchairs for mobility by adolescence. Death usually occurs prior to the age of 20 due to neoplasia or infection.

# Degenerative Disorders

A variety of progressive degenerative disorders have their onset in childhood. While most of these are not amenable to treatment, early diagnosis is important because many of these disorders are inherited and genetic counseling should be made available to families. Many of these entities fall under several different categories (degenerative, demyelinating, metabolic, or movement disorders).

## I. SPINOCEREBELLAR DEGENERATIONS

### A. Friedreich's ataxia (spinocerebellar ataxia)

1. Autosomal recessive inheritance with a prevalence of 1:48,000–100,000. The highest incidence occurs in Great Britain. The gene is located on chromosome 9.
2. Progressive degeneration of neurons primarily in the spinocerebellar tracts and the dorsal and ventral roots.
3. Onset can be as early as age 2 but is usually between the ages of 8 and 11.
4. **Features**
   a. Ataxia with a clumsy gait and frequent falls are the most common presenting features.
   b. Areflexia of the lower extremities.
   c. Dysarthria (scanning, staccato speech).
   d. Posterior column dysfunction of the lower extremities.
   e. Muscle weakness with or without hypotonia.
   f. Orthopedic deformities such as pes cavus, hammertoe, and kyphoscoliosis.
   g. Other findings include febrile convulsions (3–6 times the rate noted in the general population) and epilepsy. Diabetes mellitus can occur in up to 20% of affected patients. Other findings may include a progressive decline of fine motor skills, choreoathetoid movements, nystagmus, and cardiomyopathy.
5. **Diagnosis**
   a. Clinical history of progressive ataxia and skeletal deformities with childhood onset.
   b. **EEG** is abnormal with a generalized increase in slow waves or bursts of generalized or focal spike-waves or slow waves.
   c. **Nerve biopsy.** Fusiform and sausage-shaped axonal swellings with a decreased number of myelinated and unmyelinated fibers.
   d. **Muscle biopsy.** Small group atrophy and small angular fibers.
6. **Treatment** is primarily supportive with physical therapy and orthoses as needed. Orthopedic surgery for progressive scoliosis and foot deformities may become necessary. Follow-up with a cardiologist is essential.
7. **Outcome.** Most affected patients are unable to walk by the end of the second decade, but survival into the fourth or fifth decade is common.

### B. Olivopontocerebellar atrophies

1. Autosomal dominant inheritance in all but OPCA-II which

has a recessive inheritance pattern.

2. OPCA is a group of disorders divided into five subtypes based on clinical and pathological features. All are characterized by inferior olive, pontine, and cerebellar degeneration.

3. **Onset** is usually in adulthood except for type III, which is associated with retinal degeneration.

4. **Features** include progressive cerebellar ataxia, scanning speech, cranial nerve palsies, and extrapyramidal symptoms (rigidity, tremor). OPCA-III is associated with retinal degeneration and progressive visual loss.

5. **Diagnosis** is by clinical and family history. OPCA can be differentiated from Friedreich's ataxia by the later onset and absence of spinal cord involvement.

## C. Hereditary spastic paraplegia

1. Autosomal dominant or recessive.

2. Slowly progressive spastic paraplegia.

3. **Onset** may be in the first decade.

4. **Features**
   a. Normal milestones, sometimes with delayed onset in walking.
   b. Mild spastic paraparesis which may be incorrectly attributed to cerebral palsy. Parental evaluation may indicate that a genetic disorder is present.
   c. Upgoing toes and hyperreflexia, increased tone, and clonus in the lower extremities.
   d. Upper extremities may show mildly increased DTR.
   e. Sensation and bowel and bladder function are normal.
   f. Intelligence is normal.

5. A number of rare, complicated forms of HSP have been described with associated symptoms such as mental retardation, dementia, seizures, movement disorders, skin pigmentation, sensory neuropathies, and macular degeneration. For example, **Troyer syndrome** has been seen in Amish families with early onset of dysarthria, muscle wasting, delayed walking, and progressive spasticity.

6. **Diagnosis** of HSP is a diagnosis of exclusion. Absence of a history of prematurity or perinatal insults, and failure of progressive symptoms suggests an etiology other than cerebral palsy. Clinical examination and evaluation of parents and siblings is imperative. Important differential considerations include tethered spinal cord and tumor.

7. **Treatment** is primarily supportive with physical therapy. If the spasticity is severe, surgical treatment can be considered.

8. **Outcome** is variable. Progression to wheelchair dependency occurs in some cases, but generally not until late adulthood. In general, autosomal recessive forms tend to present earlier and have a more progressive course.

## D. Marinesco-Sjögren's syndrome

1. Rare autosomal recessive condition.

2. The hallmarks of this disorder are cerebellar ataxia, mental retardation, and bilateral cataracts.

3. No treatment is available. Cataracts can be removed surgically.

**4.** Life expectancy is normal, although afflicted individuals are significantly mentally impaired.

## II. BASAL GANGLIA DEGENERATIONS

### A. Huntington's chorea

1. Autosomal dominant inheritance with a prevalence of 5–10: 100,000. The gene for HC has been located on the short arm of chromosome 4.

2. A disorder characterized by progressive mental deterioration and the development of involuntary movements. Pathological studies have demonstrated selective loss of the GABA cells in the striatum, resulting in decreased concentrations of glutamic acid decarboxylase. Somatostatin containing cells are increased three- to fivefold.

3. **Onset** is usually between the ages of 35 and 55. About 5% of patients develop symptoms before the age of 14. The mental deterioration can begin prior to age 2. The father is the carrier in 90% of cases beginning in childhood.

4. The **features** of juvenile HC differ somewhat from adult onset HC. A progressive decline in school performance is often the first indication of the disorder. Progressive mental deterioration, behavioral disturbances, rigidity, seizures, and cerebellar signs ensue. Choreoathetosis, which is a predominant symptom in adult HC, is uncommon in childhood HC.

5. **Diagnosis** is made based on a positive parental history, clinical history, and CT or MRI evidence of caudate nucleus and cerebral cortex atrophy. However, imaging studies may not show atrophy even in symptomatic patients. PET studies showing reduced caudate glucose metabolism have been demonstrated in all symptomatic patients and one third of at-risk patients prior to the onset of their symptoms. Important differential diagnoses include juvenile Parkinson's disease, Wilson's disease, Hallervorden-Spatz syndrome, dystonia musculorum deformans, lipidoses, and Sydenham's chorea.

6. **Treatment** is not available for the dementia. Rigidity can be treated with levodopa, bromocriptine, and amantadine. Chorea may respond to haloperidol, choline, reserpine, or phenothiazines.

7. Both juvenile and adult HC are progressive with a fairly rapid decline in mental and motor function. Death usually occurs within 10–15 years after symptom onset.

### B. Juvenile Parkinson's disease (paralysis agitans)

1. In the early 1900s juvenile Parkinson's disease was seen as a sequela to encephalitis lethargica. In more recent times some sporadic and familial cases have been described.

2. Juvenile Parkinson's disease is characterized by tremor and rigidity.

3. **Diagnosis** is based on clinical features. Juvenile Parkinson's is rarely seen as a separate entity in childhood. Whenever Parkinsonian features are present in the pediatric population, other diagnoses must be considered (drug toxicity, OPCA, Wilson's disease, HC).

4. **Treatment** is symptomatic with carbidopa, levodopa, trihexyphenidyl, and other antiparkinsonian medications.

Thalamic surgery has been used successfully in the past.

**5.** The disorder is rapidly progressive. Therapy is limited by the "on-off" disturbances as seen in adults. This is characterized by the erratic appearance of periods of rigidity and bradykinesia.

**C. Hallervorden-Spatz syndrome** (pigmentary degeneration of the globus pallidus)

**1.** Rare autosomal recessive disorder.

**2.** Microscopic examination demonstrates neuronal cell loss and iron pigment deposition in the pallidum and substantia nigra. Axonal swellings forming spheroid bodies are seen throughout the basal ganglia. These are also seen in infantile neuroaxonal dystrophy, leading some authors to conclude that Hallervorden-Spatz syndrome is a juvenile form of infantile neuroaxonal dystrophy limited to the basal ganglia.

**3. Onset** is prior to the age of 15 with most cases presenting between 2 and 10 years of age.

**4. Features** include a progressive pes equinovarus causing gait disturbance, rigidity, slowing of voluntary movements, dysarthria, dystonia, choreoathetoid movements, and mental deterioration. About 30% of patients develop pigmentary retinal degeneration. Seizures are evident in some cases.

**5. Diagnosis** is based on history and imaging techniques. CT reveals bilateral high density in the basal ganglia. MRI demonstrates iron within the basal ganglia as a hypodensity in the globus pallidus on T2-weighted images. Differential diagnoses include Wilson's disease and HC.

**6. Treatment** is not available. Iron chelation, levodopa, and amantadine have been used without significant impact.

**7. Outcome** is generally death within 5–15 years after symptom onset.

**D. Dystonia musculorum deformans** (torsion dystonia)

**1.** Inheritance patterns vary. An autosomal recessive form is found predominantly among Ashkenazi Jews. Other cases are sporadic or show an autosomal dominant pattern with incomplete penetrance. In some instances, the gene has been localized to the long arm of chromosome 9.

**2.** This entity is thought to be due to a disorder in the basal ganglia, but no pathological changes have been demonstrated. Reduced levels of NE have been shown in the subthalamic nuclei, locus ceruleus, mamillary body, and the lateral and posterior hypothalamus. Conversely, increased levels of NE have been seen in the nucleus of the dorsal raphe, red nucleus, colliculi, thalamus, and septum.

**3. Onset** of this condition varies. The autosomal recessive form usually becomes symptomatic between 4 and 16 years of age and has an initial rapid decline. Other forms have a more variable time of onset.

**4. Features.** Sustained muscle contractions causing abnormal postures, twisting, and repetitive movements. It may be focal (torticollis, blepharospasm, oromandibular dystonia), segmental, or generalized. Frequently the symptoms are focal at the onset of the condition and progress to become a generalized condition.

5. **Diagnosis** is by exclusion. It is important to differentiate this condition from secondary dystonia due to drug ingestion (tricyclic antidepressants, carbamazepine, phenothiazines, phenytoin, antihistamines, lithium, ketamine, chloroquine), viral encephalitis, carbon monoxide poisoning, or craniocerebral or peripheral trauma. Other disorders that may result in dystonia and should be considered are Wilson's disease, lipidoses, and metachromatic leukodystrophy.

6. **Treatment** is aimed at diminishing the dystonia. Trihexyphenidyl, carbidopa, and tetrabenzine have all been used with some success. Diazepam, bromocriptine, and carbamazepine have been useful in some cases. Lithium in conjunction with other medications may have an additive effect. Stereotactic thalamotomy can be used in selected cases.

7. **Outcome** is based on age and site of onset. In general, early onset and onset in the legs are associated with progression to generalized dystonia. Half of all patients progress to generalized involvement within 5–10 years. The rest remain with segmental or focal dystonia. Long-term follow-up reveals that one third of patients become bedridden, one third are moderately disabled, and one third are independent but mildly disabled.

E. **Fahr's disease** (familial calcification of the basal ganglia)

1. **Fahr's disease** actually represents a group of disorders with distinct clinical and genetic patterns, all of which have in common calcification within the basal ganglia.

2. **Pathologically,** perivascular mineral deposits (pseudo-calcification) are seen within the basal ganglia.

3. **Onset** varies with the type of condition, but in some cases occurs within the first 2 years of life.

4. **Features** may include mental deterioration, choreoathetosis, microcephaly, and seizures.

5. **Diagnosis** is made with CT or MRI. When calcification is noted, underlying disorders of calcium metabolism should be ruled out (hypoparathyroidism, hyperparathyroidism, and pseudohyoparathyroidism). Toxoplasmosis, CMV, Down syndrome, Cockayne's syndrome, and tuberous sclerosis can also result in calcification of the basal ganglia.

6. **Treatment and outcome** are dependent on the underlying etiology of the condition.

## III. GRAY MATTER DEGENERATIONS

A. **Rett syndrome**

1. This sporadic disorder occurs exclusively in females. In Sweden the incidence of this disorder is 1:15,000 females.

2. Previously it was thought that this disorder was related to hyperammonemia; however, this has proven to be an inconsistent finding. Both a viral etiology and a fragile site of the Xp22 chromosome have been suggested as causes. Pathologically, diffuse cerebral atrophy, degeneration of axons in the caudate, and increased amounts of neuronal lipofusion have been described.

3. **Onset** is generally between 12 and 18 months of age but can be seen as early as 5–6 months.

4. **Features.** Developmental arrest and subsequent regression, progressive dementia, acquired microcephaly, abnormal breathing patterns (including apnea), jerking movements of the limbs and trunk, autistic behaviors, and loss of functional hand movements by age 3. The upper extremities may take on a "hand-washing" posture. Many patients go on to develop seizures and a spastic quadriparesis or paraparesis.

5. **Diagnosis** is by clinical examination.

6. There is no known treatment. Carbamazepine has been described as improving alertness even in those patients without seizures.

7. Survival can be lengthy.

## B. Infantile neuroaxonal dystrophy

1. Autosomal recessive inheritance.

2. This disorder affects axon terminals, resulting in focal axonal swelling in central and peripheral myelinated and unmyelinated axons.

3. **Onset** is usually shortly after the first 12 months of life with rapid progression to being severely handicapped by about the second year of life.

4. **Features**
   a. Motor development is abnormal with failure to progress to independent ambulation. Muscular atrophy, hypotonia, and progressive weakness develop.
   b. Increased DTR develop later in the course.
   c. Optic atrophy and ophthalmoplegia.
   d. Mental retardation.

5. **Diagnosis**
   a. Biopsy of peripheral nerves may demonstrate neuroaxonal spheroids, however these are nonspecific as they are also seen with vitamin E deficiency, Hallervorden-Spatz disease, OPCA, and Friedreich's ataxia.
   b. EEG may show generalized fast activities (over 100 μV) after age 2.
   c. EMG evidence of anterior horn cell disease.
   d. Definitive diagnosis is based on autopsy findings of large eosinophilic spheroids throughout the gray matter.

6. No treatment is available.

7. **Outcome.** Most affected children die by age 8.

## IV. WHITE MATTER

### A. Multiple sclerosis

1. MS is thought to be an immunological disorder with an underlying infectious (probably viral) etiology. There is an increased incidence of MS in individuals with HLA-B7, HLA-A3, HLA-Dw2, or HLA-DR2 tissue-type antigens. Females are affected 2–4 times as often as males. The incidence becomes greater with increasing distance from the equator. The risk of developing MS is determined by geographic location prior to puberty.

2. A demyelinating condition characterized by a chronic, remitting course. Symptoms are variable. Pathologically, there is destruction of the myelin sheath resulting in the formation of plaques of demyelination with gliosis or sclero-

sis. The plaques may be disseminated throughout the neuroaxis, but are most common in the periventricular region, the centrum semiovale, optic pathways, superior cerebellar peduncles, and the spinal cord.

**3. Onset.** MS is typically a disease of young adults, but about 1% of cases present in childhood and adolescence. Among pediatric cases, the peak onset is between 12 and 13 years. Cases presenting as early as 28 months have been reported.

**4. Features.** MS is an episodic illness, with the development of focal neurological deficits that may last weeks to months and then resolve partially or completely.

   **a.** Optic neuritis with impaired visual acuity or disturbance of ocular motility such as an internuclear ophthalmoplegia.

   **b.** Ataxia.

   **c.** Encephalopathy or mental disturbance.

   **d.** Seizures.

   **e.** Motor weakness.

   **f.** Hyperreflexia.

**5. Diagnosis**

   **a.** The clinical course is characterized by symptoms disseminated in time and within the nervous system.

   **b.** CSF obtained during an attack may show a moderate pleocytosis with predominant lymphocytes, increased protein, oligoclonal bands, and an elevated CSF IgG.

   **c.** EEG often shows diffuse or focal slowing, which while not specific may aid in distinguishing MS from other disease processes.

   **d.** MRI is very sensitive in detecting demyelinating plaques. The extent and distribution of the plaques does **not** correlate with the clinical severity of the disorder.

   **e.** Abnormalities of visual evoked responses, SSEP, and BAER can contribute to the diagnosis.

**6. Treatment** is primarily aimed at acute attacks. Prednisone (2 mg/kg/24h po) for 1 week with a taper over 1 month is effective in shortening the length of the attack. ACTH has similarly proven to be effective in decreasing the time course of an attack. Immunosuppressant therapy with azathioprine or cyclophosphamide is well described in adults but is rarely reported in children.

**7. Outcome** is variable.

**B. Diffuse cerebral sclerosis** (Schilder's disease)

   **1.** Unknown etiology. This entity is regarded by some as a form of MS seen most frequently in children.

   **2.** An entity defined as a subacute or chronic demyelinating disorder with one or more large, symmetric plaques of the centrum semiovale in the absence of other radiographic or clinical CNS or PNS lesions. Serum fatty acids are normal. Pathologically, there is extensive plaque formation in the hemispheres with sparing of subcortical white matter. Cases of necrotic, cavitating, or edematous lesions have been described.

   **3. Onset** is usually between the ages of 5 and 12.

   **4. Features.** Progressive neurological impairment in a previously healthy child. Intellectual decline, aphasia, hemiparesis, ataxia, and focal neurological deficits develop quickly.

5. **Diagnosis** can be made by MRI and clinical course. Serum very-long-chain fatty acids should be obtained to rule out adrenoleukodystrophy.

6. **Treatment** with ACTH and cyclophosphamide has been shown to improve symptoms in some cases.

7. **Outcome** is poor with complete neurological deterioration within 1–2 years after diagnosis.

## C. Alexander's disease

1. Sporadic occurrence without a familial pattern.

2. Rare condition characterized by progressive neurological deterioration. Pathologically the hallmark of this disorder is an accumulation of **Rosenthal fibers,** in particular in the periventricular, perivascular, and subpial regions. Grossly, the white matter is softened and friable with extensive demyelination. The demyelination is thought to be secondary to the primary defect of degradation of glial filaments.

3. **Onset** is typically in the first year of life, but may be delayed until later in childhood.

4. **Features.** Intellectual deterioration, seizures, spastic quadriparesis, and macrocephaly.

5. **Diagnosis** is based on clinical course, the presence of macrocephaly, and findings on imaging studies. MRI typically reveals ventriclomegaly and predominantly low attenuation of the frontal white matter bilaterally. On contrasted CT, the tips of the frontal horns may enhance. Brain biopsy is diagnostic.

6. **Treatment** is not available. Diagnosis is particularly important for prognostic considerations in that this is **not a genetic disorder** and should not influence the parents regarding future offspring.

7. Death occurs in infancy or early childhood.

## D. Pelizaeus-Merzbacher disease

1. X-linked recessive disorder primarily affecting males. Some cases of PMD in females suggest the possibility of autosomal recessive inheritance as an alternate inheritance pattern.

2. A slowly progressive disorder of myelin formation within the CNS. It has been divided into three types of disorders based on onset and patterns of abnormal myelination: type I (classical), type II (congenital), and type III (transitional). Together these are also known as the **tigroid** (tigerlike) **leukodystrophies** because of the persistence of islands of normal myelin in a perivascular distribution causing a tigroid appearance. There is relative axonal preservation in this family of disorders.

3. **Onset** is in infancy, with the congenital form appearing as early as the first few days of life.

4. **Features**

a. Prominent nystagmoid eye movements are usually evident prior to the age of 3 months.

    **b.** Oscillatory head movements with poor head control.

    **c.** Cerebellar symptoms: ataxia, intention tremor, scanning speech.

    **d.** Congenital laryngeal stridor.

    **e.** Failure to achieve developmental milestones (congenital) or progressive psychomotor deterioration (classical).

    **f.** Spasticity, optic atrophy, seizures, and involuntary movements may develop as the disease progresses.

**5.** Definitive diagnosis cannot be made until autopsy. A male with congenital stridor and nystagmoid eye movements should alert the physician to the possibility of this disorder. Imaging studies cannot differentiate this condition from other white matter diseases. On CT scan white matter is of a low attenuation with progressive atrophy. MRI shows a lack of myelination with a persistent neonatal appearance of the brain.

**6.** Treatment is not available.

**7.** The disease is progressive with occasional plateaus. The congenital form typically leads to death within the first year of life. Death in the classical form of PMD is delayed until the second to third decade.

**E. Spongy degeneration of the neuraxis** (Canavan's disease)

**1.** Autosomal recessive inheritance. This disorder is more common among Ashkenazi Jews.

**2.** A progressive disorder marked by mental deterioration and megalencephaly. Brain volume is increased. The parenchyma has a soft, gelatinous consistency. The characteristic lesion is subcortical spongiosis of the cerebral and cerebellar white matter with intramyelinic edema.

**3. Onset** is usually in the second to fourth months of life.

**4. Features**

    **a.** Failure of intellectual development.

    **b.** Optic atrophy progressing to blindness by 6–10 months of age.

    **c.** Hypotonia progressing to spasticity.

    **d.** Megalencephaly.

    **e.** Seizures.

**5. Diagnosis** is based on clinical features and course. CT and MRI reveal diffuse changes in the white matter with progressive atrophy. The serum level of N-acetylaspartic acid is elevated with associated increased urinary excretion.

**6. Treatment** is not available.

**7.** Death usually occurs prior to the second year of life, but can occur as late as the fifth.

**F. Neurolipidoses** (cerebrotendinous xanthomatosis, adrenoleukodystrophy, Wolman's disease) are discussed in Chapter 32.

**V. OTHER**

**A. Xeroderma pigmentosa**

**1.** Autosomal recessive inheritance.

**2.** A genetic disorder resulting in the absence of a gene product which excises damaged DNA and replicates beyond damaged sites of DNA. A variety of genetic subtypes have been identified, with Group A being the most common.

**3. Onset** is typically in early childhood.

**4. Features**

    **a.** Photosensitive dermatitis with erythema, freckling, keratosis, and cancers of the skin.

    **b.** Mental retardation.

    **c.** Microcephaly.

    **d.** Spinocerebellar degeneration reflected by ataxia and corticospinal signs.

    **e.** Sensorineural hearing loss.

**5. Diagnosis** can be made antenatally with cultured amniotic cells. Cultured fibroblasts from affected children demonstrate abnormal DNA repair.

**6.** The only available treatment is the avoidance of sunlight.

# Neuromuscular Disorders

A variety of neuromuscular disorders present in infancy and childhood. The diagnosis of these disorders is critical and early detection requires a high index of suspicion. Often these conditions are inherited and genetic counseling is an essential part of the management of these disorders. This chapter will review a wide range of neuromuscular disorders.

**I. MYOPATHIES.** Disorders that primarily affect the muscle fiber and/or the interstitial tissues of muscle without underlying pathology in the nervous system. Myopathies can be manifested by electrical, clinical, or pathological abnormalities. All muscular dystrophies are myopathies; however, not all myopathies are muscular dystrophies. The major forms of muscular dystrophy will be discussed in this section.

   **A. Congenital muscular dystrophy**
   1. Autosomal recessive inheritance.
   2. A rare, progressive muscular dystrophy characterized by fetal onset of profound weakness and hypotonia. The exact pathophysiology of CMD is not known. It has been suggested that the abnormalities may be due to abnormal vascular or neuronal supply to the muscle or a genetic defect of muscle surface membranes.
   3. **Features**
      a. Severe weakness and hypotonia at birth, facial weakness, dysphagia, respiratory difficulty, joint contractures (at birth or developing subsequently), congenital dislocation of the hip (25%), and spinal deformity. Pseudohypertrophy does not occur in this form of muscular dystrophy.
      b. **Arthrogryposis multiplex congenita** (contractures of two or more joints) may be present. Note that this term refers to a syndrome of "bent joints" and not to a disease entity.
      c. Intelligence is generally normal except with one of the following variations involving the central nervous system.
         (1) **Fukuyama congenital muscular dystrophy** is a syndrome of CMD with cerebellar and cerebral gyral abnormalities (polymicrogyria, pachygyria, agyria). Profound mental retardation (IQ 30–50), febrile and afebrile seizures, and serum CPK levels 10–50 times normal are common in these patients.
         (2) **Cerebro-ocular dysplasia (Walker-Warburg syndrome).** CMD with associated gyral abnormalities (polymicrogyria, pachygyria, agyria), hydrocephalus and ocular abnormalities.
   4. **Diagnosis**
      a. **EMG.** Reduced amplitudes and mean durations with increased polyphasia (Table 16-1).
      b. **CPK.** Usually elevated 2.5–7 times normal.

**Table 16-1. Characteristic EMG findings**

| Type | EMG findings |
|------|--------------|
| Myopathy | Decreased amplitude and duration of motor unit potentials. Numerous polyphasic potentials. |
| Myotonia | Repetitive electrical potentials (up to 100/sec) that decrease over time. Characteristic "dive-bomber" sound. |
| Neuromuscular junction | Abnormal fluctuations in the size and shape of motor unit potentials with movement. Progressive decrements of muscle action potential amplitude with stimulation. Increased jitter (prolonged interpotential interval) between two muscle fibers in an activated motor unit. |

    **c. Muscle biopsy** shows islands of rounded, variably sized muscle fibers surrounded by fat and connective tissue which have replaced muscle fibers.

    **d. MRI.** Abnormalities of the gyri or white matter in those patients with CNS involvement.

  **5. Treatment** is primarily supportive. Physical therapy to prevent the development of contractures and maximize muscle strength should be instituted early. Spinal deformities may require surgical correction.

  **6. Outcome.** Often there is a history of decreased fetal movements in utero. Postnatally the course varies. It may be nonprogressive or demonstrate slow improvement. Other patients progress to death.

**B. Duchenne muscular dystrophy**

  **1.** X-linked recessive inherited disorder primarily affecting males, with one third of cases due to new mutations. The gene has been localized to the small arm of chromosome X (Xp21). The protein product of the normal gene, dystrophin, is reduced to 3% of normal in most children with DMD. The incidence of this disorder is reported as 1:3000–8000 males.

  **2.** A pseudohypertrophic form of muscular dystrophy that progresses fairly rapidly, affecting proximal muscles more than distal muscles and the pelvic girdle muscles before the shoulder girdle muscles. Duchenne muscular dystrophy is the most common form of muscular dystrophy.

  **3. Onset** is typically between the ages of 3 and 6. Often this is characterized by an insidious difficulty climbing stairs and arising from the floor, with a fairly rapid progression of muscular weakness to the inability to walk by age 12.

  **4. Features**

    **a.** Muscular weakness that is more pronounced proximally. Involvement of the pelvic girdle usually precedes involvement of the shoulder girdle. Use of the **Gowers' maneu-ver** to rise from a seated position on the floor to a standing position, by "climbing" up the legs using the arms, may be noted early on. The ability to jump or hop is significantly impaired or absent. The gait is slow, awkward, waddling, and unsteady. Heel-cord contractures lead to toe-walking.

   **b.** DTR at the knee may be absent early on, but are preserved at the ankles, helping to distinguish DMD from denervating disorders.

   **c.** Sensory examination is normal.

   **d.** Pseudohypertrophy of the calf muscles with fat and connective tissue.

   **e.** Mental retardation. The mean IQ is 85 with one third of patients having an IQ below 75. The severity of mental retardation is not related to the severity of physical weakness.

   **f.** Cardiomyopathy with tachycardia and heart failure may be fatal.

   **g.** Skeletal malformations: scoliosis, lumbar lordosis, kyphosis, and rarefaction and narrowing of long bones.

   **h.** Symptoms of smooth muscle dysfunction: swallowing disturbance, vomiting, abdominal distention, and diarrhea.

   **i.** Female carriers may be asymptomatic or display mild weakness of the pelvic musculature and pseudo-hypertrophy.

**5. Diagnosis**

   **a. Clinical features.** The time from onset of first symptoms to diagnosis may be as long as 2.5 years.

   **b. EMG.** Myopathic changes (Table 16-1).

   **c. CPK** levels are markedly elevated.

   **d. Muscle biopsy** contributes to a diagnosis but findings are not pathognomic. Findings include variable muscle fiber diameter, necrosis and cellular infiltration, proliferation of interstitial connective tissue, and evidence of fiber regeneration.

   **e. ECG abnormalities.** Tall R-waves in the right precordial leads and deep Q-waves in all limb leads.

**6. Treatment** is primarily supportive. Surgical intervention should be delayed as long as possible. Physical therapy to minimize contractures is imperative. A weight control program can help maximize ambulatory time. When the patient is wheelchair-bound, early bracing programs can help prevent further spinal deformity and ultimately bedridden status. Parents should be encouraged to help afflicted children develop interests in reading, painting, or similar activities that require little physical activity. Prevention through genetic counseling is important. Obviously, it is imperative to distinguish between the X-linked form of inheritance and a new mutation. Most carriers have elevated CPK levels and some degree of myopathy.

**7. Outcome.** Muscular weakness is progressive and the ability to ambulate is usually lost in early adolescence. Death occurs in the late second or early third decade due to infection, respiratory compromise, or cardiac failure.

**C. X-linked recessive muscular dystrophy** (Becker's muscular dystrophy)

1. Sex-linked recessive inheritance. The Becker's form of muscular dystrophy has a much more benign course. It is present in approximately 10% of patients with sex-linked recessive muscular dystrophy. Dystrophin is present in normal amounts, but with an abnormal configuration (see sec. I. B. 1).

2. A more benign, gradually progressive loss of muscle strength in a pattern similar to that seen with DMD.

3. **Onset** is typically between the ages of 4 and 25.

4. **Features.** This disorder is similar to DMD, but is usually later in onset and has a much more benign course, with ambulatory capacity retained sometimes to 25 years after diagnosis. Pseudohypertrophy of the calf muscles may make it difficult to distinguish from DMD early on. Ankle reflexes are often absent. Some degree of mental retardation may occur. Cardiac involvement is uncommon (< 15% of cases).

5. **Diagnosis.** Distinguishing Becker's muscular dystrophy from DMD can be difficult and ultimately may be based on the rate of progression. Clinical findings, elevated CPK (may be as high as DMD), myopathic changes on EMG, and muscle biopsy demonstrate changes similar to those seen in DMD.

6. **Treatment** is supportive as with DMD.

7. **Outcome.** Slow progression of muscular weakness leads to loss of ambulation sometimes as late as 25 years after the onset.

**D. Facioscapulohumeral muscular dystrophy** (Landouzy-Dejerine dystrophy)

1. Autosomal dominant inheritance and a large number of sporadic cases.

2. A slowly progressive muscular dystrophy characterized by facial weakness in addition to shoulder girdle weakness and upper limb weakness.

3. **Onset** is usually between the ages of 7 and 12, but earlier onset has been reported.

4. **Features**

   a. Facial weakness, weakness of the orbicularis oculi with inability to close the eyes (may sleep with eyes open), and impaired sucking. Weakness may be asymmetrical.

   b. Progressive weakness of the shoulder girdle with winging of the scapulae. Limb musculature usually becomes involved later in the course.

   c. Skeletal abnormalities, contractures, and cardiac involvement are rarely seen.

   d. Retinal vascular abnormalities demonstrated by fluorescence angiography may be identified in up to 75% of cases.

5. **Diagnosis.** Normal to raised CPK levels and myopathic changes on EMG. Results from muscle biopsies are variable. The most severe changes have been noted in younger

patients who display significant endomysial fibrosis around variably hypertrophic and atrophic fibers. Biopsies in older children show generalized fiber hypertrophy and foci of inflammatory cells.

6. **Treatment** is supportive. The same guidelines outlined for DMD apply to FSHMD.

7. **Outcome.** FSHMD is a slowly progressive disorder that is associated with a normal life span.

## E. Limb-girdle muscular dystrophy

1. This is actually a group of related disorders with variable inheritance. Autosomal recessive inheritance is most common, but sporadic and dominant patterns occur as well.

2. This group of disorders has a variable rate of progression and is characterized by initial involvement of the pelvic or shoulder girdle.

3. **Onset** is highly variable, with some forms beginning in the first decade, and others presenting as late as the second or third decades.

4. **Features.** Variably progressive weakness starting in the shoulder or pelvic girdle. The heart is usually not involved and mental function remains normal. Only 30% of patients develop pseudohypertrophy.

5. **Diagnosis** is based on clinical features and muscle biopsy that typically reveals fiber hypertrophy and increased endomysial connective tissue. CPK, EMG, and NCV help rule out other disorders but have no specific features in this set of disorders.

6. **Treatment** is supportive.

7. **Outcome** is variable, but overall the course is much more benign than that seen with DMD.

## F. Emery-Dreifuss muscular dystrophy

1. Rare, X-linked disorder localized to the long arm of the X-chromosome (Xq28).

2. A slowly progressive weakness predominantly involving the biceps, triceps, and peroneal muscles with associated cardiac conduction abnormalities.

3. **Onset** is between 5 and 15 years of age.

4. **Features**
   a. Weakness is predominantly in the biceps, triceps, and distal musculature of the legs.
   b. Early contractures of the posterior cervical muscles, elbows, and Achilles tendon.
   c. Cardiac arrhythmias are often fatal.
   d. Lack of muscular hypertrophy.
   e. Nocturnal hypoventilation.

5. **Diagnosis** is based on clinical features, in particular the early contractures and cardiac arrhythmias. Muscle biopsy and EMG show mixed patterns (neurogenic and/or myopathic).

6. **Treatment** is supportive. Nocturnal hypoventilation can be managed with tracheotomy and nighttime ventilatory support. Cardiac arrhythmias may require placement of a permanent pacemaker.

7. **Outcome** is variable. The progression is slow, with some

patients stabilizing in adulthood and others progressing to be wheelchair-bound or bedridden. Cardiac arrhythmias are often fatal.

### G. Central core disease

1. Autosomal dominant inheritance.
2. Mild, nonprogressive muscular weakness.
3. **Onset** is early, usually in infancy.
4. **Features.** Hypotonia, mild, nonprogressive weakness, muscle contractures, cardiac abnormalities, congenital dislocation of the hip, and other skeletal abnormalities (pes cavus, kyphoscoliosis). Many of those afflicted have a tendency toward **malignant hyperthermia.**
5. **Diagnosis.** Muscle biopsy using special techniques to demonstrate mitochondrial enzyme activity or phosphorylase activity reveals central areas without activity, suggesting a loss of mitochondria. Type I fiber predominance is also noted.
6. **Treatment** is supportive.
7. **Outcome** is generally good. Those afflicted with central core disease may note only mild weakness. Some children are more severely afflicted with severe scoliosis and more profound weakness.

### H. Nemaline myopathy

1. Inheritance of this disorder may be through either an autosomal dominant pattern with variable penetrance or an autosomal recessive pattern.
2. Myopathy characterized by hypotonia and progressive respiratory difficulties.
3. **Onset** is ordinarily in the first months of life, but some adult-onset forms exist.
4. **Features.** Hypotonia, weakness, loss of muscle bulk, facial weakness, and feeding difficulties with or without respiratory failure. Often patients display skeletal abnormalities (kyphoscoliosis, pes cavus, arched palate).
5. **Diagnosis** is by muscle biopsy that shows pathognomonic red-staining threadlike structures within muscle fibers.
6. **Treatment** is supportive.
7. **Outcome.** The course varies. The worst prognosis is associated with cases of neonatal onset of profound weakness and respiratory compromise ultimately leading to early death. More benign courses may have a neonatal onset or adult onset of less profound weakness. Cases may be nonprogressive or slowly progressive with skeletal abnormalities developing over time.

### I. Myotubular myopathy (centrotubular myopathy)

1. Likely autosomal dominant inheritance with variable penetrance.
2. Nonprogressive to slowly progressive weakness of the limbs with frequent involvement of the extraocular muscles and ptosis. The name is based on the pathological appearance of the muscle, which is similar to the myotubules of fetal muscle.
3. **Onset** is usually in infancy, but can be in late childhood. A more severe X-linked recessive form has been reported with onset in the neonatal period and is associated with neonatal

asphyxia. In some cases, evidence for decreased fetal movement and hydramnios suggest a prenatal onset.

4. **Features.** Weakness of the limbs, loss of DTR, ptosis, and external ophthalmoplegia.

5. **Diagnosis** is based on clinical exam and muscle biopsy that shows persistence of fetal myotubules, a predominance of type I fibers, and increased central staining for oxidative enzymes.

6. **Treatment** is supportive.

7. **Outcome** is based on the severity of the disease, with patients with the most severe cases dying in infancy.

## J. Congenital fiber-type disproportion

1. Inheritance is variable, with the majority of cases occurring sporadically. There are some cases which show autosomal dominant inheritance patterns.

2. This group of muscle diseases has in common a histological picture of type I fibers smaller than type II fibers. This characteristic feature has been noted in infants with fetal alcohol syndrome and myotonic dystrophy as well as other disorders.

3. **Onset** is generally in infancy, but may be delayed until early childhood.

4. **Features.** Hypotonia, congenital dislocation of the hip, and joint contractures. The degree of weakness is variable and usually peaks by the age of 2. In some cases kyphoscoliosis develops.

5. **Diagnosis** is by muscle biopsy showing the characteristic type I fibers smaller than type II fibers.

6. **Treatment** with an aggressive physical therapy program diminishes the incidence of contractures.

7. **Outcome** is usually favorable, except in those cases with severe respiratory compromise.

## K. Mitochondrial (respiratory chain) myopathies

1. Most appear to be transmitted by autosomal recessive patterns, but inheritance patterns are not entirely clear. Inheritance appears to be primarily through maternal sources because only small amounts of paternal mitochondria are transmitted at the time of fertilization of the ovum.

2. These disorders are due to defects in the respiratory chain that is located on the inner mitochondrial membrane. It is composed of four protein complexes: complex I (NADH–coenzyme Q reductase), complex II (succinate–coenzyme Q reductase), complex III (reduced coenzyme Q–cytochrome $c$ reductase), and complex IV (cytochrome $c$ oxidase).

3. **Onset** can be anytime from birth to adulthood.

4. **Features.** Exercise intolerance with or without external ophthalmoplegia, dementia, retinitis pigmentosa, neuropathy, deafness, seizures, involuntary movements, and ataxia. Half of all patients develop exercise intolerance and three quarters can be expected to develop an ophthalmoplegia.

5. **Diagnosis** is by clinical presentation. Children with exercise intolerance and ophthalmoplegia should be evaluated with a Tensilon test to distinguish between myasthenia gravis and mitochondrial myopathies. Glucose-lactate tol-

erance testing in mitochondrial myopathies reveals lactic acidosis. Muscle biopsy reveals mitochondrial clumping known as "ragged red fibers," as demonstrated by using the modified Gomori trichrome reaction.

6. **Treatment.** None has been found to be effective.

7. **Outcome** is variable and based on the severity of the symptoms. In some cases a fatal lactic acidosis develops shortly after birth.

L. **Restricted myopathies.** A variety of myopathies with limited motor involvement have been described. Some of these are briefly listed and described below.

1. **Congenital ptosis** is unilateral in 70% of cases and bilateral in the remaining 30%.

2. **Congenital third nerve palsy** is usually unilateral with or without pupillary involvement. Most cases are idiopathic, but underlying causes (tumor, aneurysm) should be ruled out.

3. **Duane's retraction syndrome.** Fibrosis of one or both lateral rectus muscles. On attempted adduction the globe is retracted and elevated.

4. **Möbius' syndrome.** Congenital bilateral lower motor neuron facial weakness. It may be associated with external ophthalmoplegias, lower cranial nerve palsies (IX, X, XI, XII) and skeletal deformities (arthrogryposis, syndactyly). If significant lower cranial nerve dysfunction is present, there may be feeding and respiratory difficulties.

M. **Inflammatory myopathies**

1. **Polymyositis.** Hypotonia, weakness, poor suck, and a weak cry. Marked elevations in CPK, elevated ESR, and inflammatory changes on muscle biopsy suggest this diagnosis. Treatment with steroids may be worthwhile.

2. **Dermatomyositis** includes, in addition to features of polymyositis, a heliotrope rash on the eyelids, a facial butterfly rash, and scaly rashes of the extremities. Histologically, arteritis is present. The gastrointestinal system may be affected as manifested by abdominal pain, discomfort, and hemorrhage.

3. **Minimal change myopathy** encompasses any clinically detected congenital myopathy that does not demonstrate significant abnormalities of CPK, EMG, or muscle fibers. These patients tend to improve over time and carry a good prognosis.

N. **Endocrine myopathies.** Hyperadrenalism, hypoadrenalism, hyperparathyroidism, hypoparathyroidism, hyperthyroidism, and hypothyroidism can all be associated with proximal limb weakness usually greater in the legs than the arms. DTR are normal or diminished. Workup with appropriate endocrine studies based on other clinical information should be performed. Treatment of the underlying disorder is usually associated with an improvement in myopathic symptoms.

II. **MYOTONIC DISORDERS.** Myotonic disorders are characterized by persistent active contraction of the muscle after termination of a stimulus or voluntary movement. Exposure to the cold can aggravate myotonia, and repetitive movement may decrease myotonia. EMG characteristics are shown in Table 16-1.

A. **Congenital myotonic dystrophy** (Steinhart's syndrome)
   1. Autosomal dominant inheritance invariably of maternal origin for reasons that are not clear. This is the most common myopathic disorder of infancy with an incidence of 13.5:100,000.
   2. **Pathophysiology.** Disturbed or arrested maturation of muscles probably due to abnormal innervation of developing muscles.
   3. **Features**
      a. Hypotonia, weakness, respiratory and feeding difficulties, facial diplegia, "tented" upper lip, areflexia, atrophy, and delayed motor development. Myotonia is not usually demonstrable until late in infancy.
      b. Impaired gastric motility.
      c. Arthrogryposis.
      d. Impaired intellect (IQ 50–65).
      e. Cardiac dysfunction, cataracts, balding, and facial and gonadal atrophy become evident with age.
   4. **Clinical course.** Often there is a history of hydramnios during pregnancy, suggesting an in utero abnormality of swallowing. Symptoms are usually evident in the initial hours or days of life. Death in the neonatal period occurs in 50% of cases. Only 20% of children survive to adolescence or adulthood. Survivors of infancy in general have some improvement in respiratory and feeding dysfunction. The majority of these survivors has significant impairment of gastrointestinal function with chronic diarrhea and abdominal pain.
   5. **Diagnosis**
      a. Clinical examination.
      b. Features of myotonic dystrophy in the mother (facial diparesis, myotonia, cataracts).
      c. EMG. Myotonic changes (Table 16-1).
      d. CPK is normal.
   6. **Treatment**
      a. **Genetic counseling.** Antenatal amniocentesis detects the gene for secretor status in 15% of cases. Myopathic women who have previously had an affected neonate have nearly a 30% chance of giving birth to another affected newborn. Myopathic women who have previously given birth to a child with late-onset disease have only a 5% chance of giving birth to another affected newborn. Late-onset disease in children born to myopathic women occurs in 30% of cases.
      b. **Treatment** is supportive in terms of respiratory care and nutritional support. Metoclopramide has been used with some success in infants with very poor gastric motility.

B. **Myotonica congenita** (Thomsen's disease)
   1. Usually transmitted in an autosomal dominant manner, but there have been some reports of autosomal recessive

inheritance.

2. Characterized by myotonia without mental or endocrine dysfunction.

3. **Onset** is typically in infancy, but may be delayed until the second decade.

4. **Features**

   a. Early in infancy feeding difficulties and impaired eyelid opening can be noticeable.

   b. Diffuse muscular hypertrophy ("infant Hercules").

   c. Myotonia is increased with commencement of movement and may be improved with continued activity.

5. **Diagnosis** is based on clinical findings and myopathic changes on EMG (parents should be investigated as well). Muscle biopsy is usually nonspecific, although an abnormal distribution of ATPase-staining fibers has been noted. The CPK level is normal.

6. **Treatment** is supportive with physical therapy as needed.

7. **Outcome.** The myotonia usually improves with age.

C. **Paramyotonia congenita** (Eulenburg disease)

   1. Dominant inheritance.

   2. Myotonia on exposure to the cold and episodic flaccid paralysis.

   3. **Onset** is usually in infancy or early childhood.

   4. **Features.** Myotonia brought on by the cold and increasing with prolonged exercise. Periods of flaccid paralysis occur and muscle wasting may develop. An association with weakness and increased serum potassium has been noted in some cases, suggesting a connection with hyperkalemic periodic paralysis.

   5. **Diagnosis** is based primarily on history.

   6. **Treatment** is supportive, with avoidance of the cold.

D. **Schwartz-Jampel syndrome** (chondrodystrophic myotonia)

   1. Rare, recessively inherited disorder.

   2. Myotonia causing a "pinched" appearance of the face.

   3. **Onset** may be noted early in infancy.

   4. **Features.** Generalized myopathy, myotonia with involvement of the facial musculature causing blepharospasm and mouth puckering, vertebral anomalies, skeletal deformities, short stature, and normal intelligence.

   5. **Diagnosis** is by clinical symptoms and EMG evidence of myotonia (Table 16-1).

   6. **Treatment** involves physical therapy and orthopedic surgery if necessary. Procainamide can be used to treat severe myotonia.

E. **Periodic paralyses** are a group of uncommon disorders characterized by periodic, temporary paralysis with associated loss of DTR. Between episodes, patients are normal. These are transmitted by autosomal dominant inheritance patterns. Potassium and sodium metabolism have been found to be important in these disorders. Diagnosis is based on a positive family history and response to therapy.

   1. **Hypokalemic periodic paralysis**

      a. Affects males 3 times more often than females, with most

    episodes occurring between the ages of 7 and 21.

    **b.** Weakness is most pronounced in the lower limbs, but can progress to affect the respiratory and bulbar musculature.

    **c.** Symptoms typically develop with serum potassium concentrations of less than 3 mEq/L.

    **d.** Attacks are precipitated by a large carbohydrate meal, rest after exercise, exposure to cold, and administration of insulin, ACTH, or mineralocorticoids.

    **e.** The duration of the attack is from 6–24 hours.

    **f. Treatment**

        **(1)** Prevention with a diet high in potassium and low in sodium and carbohydrates. Potassium supplements may be required.

        **(2)** Acute attacks are treated with oral or intravenous potassium and supportive therapy as indicated.

    **g. Outcome.** Death related to respiratory involvement may occur. Progressive muscular atrophy can develop.

**2. Normokalemic periodic paralysis.** Transient periods of severe weakness that may persist for days to weeks, associated with a normal serum potassium. Treatment with oral sodium supplements can improve the weakness.

**3. Hyperkalemic periodic paralysis**

    **a.** Presents in the first decade of life and has no gender prevalence.

    **b.** Weakness is most pronounced in the pelvic musculature but can become more generalized.

    **c.** Attacks usually last around 1 hour and occur as often as weekly. During an attack, the serum potassium is noted to be higher than normal.

    **d.** Treatment is usually unnecessary.

## III. DISORDERS OF NEUROMUSCULAR TRANSMISSION

    **A. Myasthenia gravis.** Several forms of myasthenia gravis and myasthenic syndromes have been described. In general, this is a condition associated with fatigue of voluntary muscles due to defective neuromuscular transmission. In most cases this has been related to a loss of functional acetylcholine receptors. In some forms of myasthenia this is due to an autoimmune process.

    **1. Transient neonatal myasthenia** occurs in 10–15% of infants born to mothers with myasthenia gravis. Symptoms of hypotonia and bulbar weakness (feeding difficulty, weak cry) are usually evident within the first 3 days of life and persist no longer than 8 weeks. The diagnosis is made based on maternal history and demonstration of increased serum levels of AChRP antibodies. Anticholinesterase medications and exchange transfusion can be instituted in severe cases. This is a transitory condition and does not develop into myasthenia.

    **2. Familial infantile myasthenia** is thought to be inherited in an autosomal recessive pattern. It is characterized by generalized hypotonia, feeding difficulties, and severe respiratory insufficiency with onset at birth. Respiratory difficulties may be sufficiently severe as to require mechanical ventilation. Diagnosis can be made by Tensilon test and with nerve stimulation studies demonstrating a progressive decrement in the amplitude of successive motor unit potentials. Serum AChRP antibodies are not elevated. This syndrome is not thought to have an autoimmune basis. Long-term treatment with anticholinesterase drugs is necessary.

3. **Congenital myasthenia gravis** occurs in infants born to mothers without myasthenia. A variety of syndromes have been recognized. The underlying causes are variable and include congenital deficiency of end-plate acetylcholinesterase, abnormal acetylcholine-ion channels, acetylcholine receptor deficiencies, and defective acetylcholine resynthesis and mobilization. Clinically, congenital myasthenia gravis varies depending on the underlying pathophysiology. In general, there is a pattern of persistent weakness, ptosis, and ophthalmoparesis beginning in the newborn period. Treatment varies according to the underlying defect. Symptoms usually persist into adulthood.

4. **Juvenile myasthenia gravis** is similar to the myasthenia gravis seen in adults. It is characterized by waxing and waning of abnormal fatigability of voluntary muscles. Females are affected 2–6 times as often as males. Symptoms develop after 6 months of age, most commonly in the second decade. Presenting symptoms include ptosis, ophthalmoplegia, facial weakness, dysphonia, extremity weakness, respiratory difficulties, and chewing difficulties. As with the adult form, there is usually an increased serum concentration of AChRP antibodies suggesting an autoimmune basis. The diagnosis is confirmed by Tensilon test and EMG evidence of a decrement in the amplitude of successive action potentials. Treatment options include anticholinesterase drugs, immunosuppressive therapy, plasma exchange, and thymectomy.

B. **Toxins**
1. *Clostridium tetani*
   a. Infection of a wound with *C. tetani* results in tetanus. In infants, the umbilical cord may be a site of entry.
   b. *Clostridium tetani* spores flourish in anaerobic conditions and produce the neurotoxin **tetanospasmin,** which affects the nervous system by blocking the release of acetylcholine from nerve terminals and selective blockage of inhibitory synapses in the CNS.
   c. **Onset** ranges from 24 hours to 3 weeks after introduction of the tetanus bacilli into a wound.
   d. **Features.** Pain and stiffness of the back and neck progress to severe spasm. Cranial nerve function may become impaired (cephalic tetanus). Significant autonomic symptoms can develop, including sweating, tachycardia, arrhythmias, hypertension, and fever. Respiratory function can become compromised.
   e. **Diagnosis** is based on a history of injury and the clinical exam.
   f. **Treatment.** The best treatment is prevention through active immunization. However, once tetanus has devel-

oped, intensive supportive treatment includes debridement of infected tissue, antibiotics, and administration of antitoxin to neutralize toxin that has not become fixed in tissues. Human hyperimmune globulin (30–300 U/kg IM) should be administered in a timely fashion. Spasms may require therapy with diazepam.

**g. Outcome.** With aggressive early management and supportive care, the outcome can be quite favorable.

**2.** *Clostridium botulinum*

**a.** Entry into the body is usually through the ingestion of contaminated food (e.g., raw honey) or through wounds infected with *C. botulinum*.

**b.** The toxin released by *C. botulinum* irreversibly blocks acetylcholine release at the neuromuscular junction, causing an acute descending flaccid paralysis.

**c. Onset** of symptoms is typically within 18–36 hours after ingestion of contaminated food, but can be sooner.

**d. Features.** Common presenting symptoms include dizziness, diploplia, blurred vision, and bulbar dysfunction (dysphagia, dysarthria). There is a common pattern of descending involvement with respiratory dysfunction and a flaccid paralysis. The pupillary reflex is usually intact. The sensory system is not affected.

**e. Diagnosis** is based on recovery of the toxin in stool or isolation of the organism.

**f. Treatment.** Administration of **botulism antitoxin trivalent** as soon as possible following exposure may minimize symptoms. Respiratory failure is common and requires ventilatory support until recovery. If swallowing is impaired, tube feeding may be necessary.

**g. Outcome.** Even the most severely afflicted patients will have a complete recovery if adequately supported. Complete recovery may take weeks to months.

**3. Tick paralysis** can develop after a bite by a variety of ticks. The presentation is a rapidly progressive symmetric, flaccid paralysis which may involve the facial musculature, areflexia, and numbness or tingling of the extremities and face. CSF protein is normal as compared with the elevated protein seen in GBS. Removal of the tick is therapeutic and associated with a good recovery.

## IV. ANTERIOR HORN CELL DISORDERS

**A. Type 1 spinal muscular atrophy** (Werdnig-Hoffmann disease)

**1.** Autosomal recessive inheritance.

**2.** A syndrome of anterior horn cell degeneration characterized by profound hypotonia and reduced motor strength.

**3. Onset** is in the newborn period in 40% of cases with 80% of cases becoming apparent before 9 months of age. Frequently there is a history of decreased fetal movement in the last trimester.

**4. Features**

**a.** Profound weakness, hypotonia, and areflexia.

**b.** Sensation, sphincter function, and mentation are normal.

**c.** As the disease progresses, the bulbar musculature often becomes involved and respiratory difficulty may develop.

**d.** Fasciculations and tongue atrophy develop in approximately one third of patients.

**e.** Despite the profound weakness, the infant appears alert and bright-eyed.

**5. Diagnosis**

**a.** History and clinical examination.

**b.** CPK is normal.

**c.** **EMG** can demonstrate spontaneous, regular discharges at 5–15 seconds. Fibrillations and rest fasciculations are usually apparent.

**d.** **Muscle biopsy** demonstrates changes consistent with denervation.

**e.** Chest radiographs often demonstrate deformities and thin ribs related to congenital neuromuscular dysfunction.

**6. Treatment** is supportive. Tube feeding and careful pulmonary toilet are essential. The issue of ventilatory support in this rapidly progressive disorder is an ethical dilemma.

**7. Outcome.** In general, early onset is associated with a poor prognosis. Sixty percent of afflicted children die by the age of 2, and 80% by the age of 4.

**B. Type 2 spinal muscular atrophy**

**1.** Autosomal dominant, recessive, and apparently nongenetic cases have been reported.

**2.** A more benign form of anterior horn cell degeneration with hypotonia and weakness.

**3. Onset** of symptoms is between 3 and 15 months of age with a mean of 6 months.

**4. Features.** Weakness, hypotonia, areflexia, and skeletal malformations. A tremor of the upper extremities helps distinguish this condition. Bulbar function is usually not impaired, but respiratory function can become compromised. Intelligence is normal.

**5. Diagnosis**

**a.** History and clinical exam.

**b.** Creatinine kinase is increased fivefold in approximately half of affected patients.

**c.** **EMG** findings of fibrillations and fasciculations.

**6. Treatment** is supportive. Bracing for skeletal malformations may become necessary.

**7. Outcome** is variable. Some patients survive into adolescence.

**C. Late onset juvenile spinal muscular atrophy** (Kugelberg-Welander disease)

**1.** Variable genetic patterns (autosomal recessive, dominant, and X-linked) of inheritance have been reported.

**2.** A milder and later presenting form of anterior horn degeneration associated with predominantly proximal motor weakness.

**3. Onset** is as early as age 2, but as late as adulthood.

**4. Features.** Proximal motor weakness, impaired joint mobility, and in some cases fasciculations.

**5. Diagnosis** is based on history, clinical examination, EMG evidence of fasciculations, and muscle biopsy demonstrating denervation changes.

    **6. Treatment** is supportive. Bracing or orthopedic surgery may be required to maintain mobility.

    **7. Outcome** is variable based on age of onset and degree of involvement, but in general this is a more benign and chronic form of spinal muscular atrophy associated with long-term survival.

## V. DRUG-INDUCED MYOPATHIC SYNDROMES

### A. Malignant hyperthermia

1. Autosomal dominant inheritance with variable penetrance. The incidence of malignant hyperthermia with general anesthesia is 1:10,000.

2. A dramatic elevation in body temperature and muscular rigidity triggered by the administration of certain inhalational anesthetic agents.

3. This syndrome is usually precipitated by general anesthesia in susceptible individuals. A family history of elevated temperature with general anesthetics should alert the clinician to the possibility of malignant hyperthermia.

4. **Features.** Administration of an anesthetic agent (in particular, halothane or suxamethonium) or succinylcholine precipitates this syndrome.

    a. A rapid elevation of body temperature, up to $2^0$ C per hour.

    b. Tachycardia and tachypnea.

    c. Muscular rigidity and muscular fasciculations.

    d. Progressive metabolic acidosis.

5. **Diagnosis** is based on the clinical reaction to an anesthetic. Serum CPK rises significantly.

6. **Treatment.** There is no reliable screening measure for this condition. A family history of hyperthermia with anesthesia should be inquired about prior to general anesthesia.

    a. **Prophylaxis** for susceptible patients requiring surgery: dantrolene sodium 4–8 mg/kg/24h divided q6h PO for 1–2 days prior to surgery with the last dose 4 hours prior to induction.

    b. **Acute treatment**

      (1) Discontinue anesthesia.

      (2) Dantrolene sodium 1 mg/kg IV and repeat every 5–10 minutes to a maximum dose of 10 mg/kg.

      (3) Body cooling and treatment of the metabolic acidosis with intravenous sodium bicarbonate.

7. **Outcome.** The mortality rate is approximately 65%.

### B. Neuroleptic malignant syndrome

1. The development of hyperthermia, muscular rigidity, autonomic dysfunction (hypertension, fever), and change in consciousness related to the therapeutic (not toxic) use of some neuroleptic drugs (butyrophenones, thioxanthenes, phenothiazenes).

2. This syndrome develops predominantly in young males. Children with epilepsy, mental retardation, and cerebral palsy also have an increased incidence of neuroleptic malignant syndrome.

3. **Treatment** is withdrawal of the responsible drug. Bromocriptine can be administered. Supportive care may be necessary for blood pressure control and respiratory

impairment.
4. **Outcome.** Cessation of medication usually results in complete recovery in 3–5 days. There is a 20% mortality rate, most often due to respiratory collapse.

# Craniosynostosis

The term craniosynostosis refers to a group of disorders characterized by the premature closure of one or several of the cranial sutures. The name is derived from the involved suture. These are discussed below, along with several syndromes in which craniosynostosis is a predominant feature.

## I. GENERAL
- **A.** The cranial sutures are present to accommodate the rapid brain growth which occurs in infancy. The weight of the brain increases threefold in the first year of life.
- **B.** In cases of multiple suture involvement or pansynostosis, the surgical treatment of craniosynostosis is aimed at the prevention of increased ICP.
- **C.** The incidence of craniosynostosis is in the range of 1:1900 live births. There is a male preponderance in craniosynostosis with 63% of overall cases occurring in males. This is even higher in scaphocephaly and trigonocephaly, with 75–80% of the cases occurring in males.
- **D.** There is no proof that single-suture synostosis affects cognitive function. However, there are some reports of increased ICP with single-suture synostosis.

## II. ETIOLOGY.
Craniosynostosis was first recognized and named by Virchow in 1851. He noted that premature synostosis of a cranial suture restricts perpendicular growth and exaggerates parallel growth (with respect to the fused suture). Since then a number of theories have been proposed to explain this premature fusion.
- **A.** Moss set forth one of the earliest theories, which suggested that craniosynostosis occurred as a result of a primary malformation of the cranial base. This abnormality in turn alters the tensile force of evolving dural fiber tracts, resulting in premature synostosis of the sutures.
- **B.** More recently, it has been proposed that craniosynostosis results from a failure of bony microspicules bridging the sutures to fracture during development, thus forming a bridge for deposition of bone.
- **C.** Another proposition is that premature fusion of a suture leads to restricted bone plates and abnormal bony deposition.
- **D.** Other suggested causes include intrauterine infection, intrauterine constraint, birth trauma, and metabolic abnormalities (rickets, idiopathic hypercalcemia, hypophosphatemia, hyperthyroidism, mucopolysaccharidosis, polycythemia vera, sickle cell disease, thalassemia major, and ataxia-telangiectasia).

## III. DIAGNOSIS AND TREATMENT
- **A.** True craniosynostosis, which is a malformation, must be differentiated from deformation as a result of intrauterine constraint. Deformation will improve with time and corrective positioning. On the contrary, a malformation will worsen with time.

**B.** The diagnosis of craniosynostosis is often made with a **visual inspection** of the patient. Abnormal growth occurs in a predictable fashion, with failure of skull growth perpendicular to the involved suture and exaggerated growth parallel to the involved suture.

**C.** **Plain radiographs** are generally diagnostic. More sophisticated radiographic studies such as fluoroscopy or 3-D CT may be useful.

**D.** There may be signs of **elevated ICP** on plain radiographs, since 40% of patients with multiple suture involvement have been reported to have increased pressure. With single suture synostosis this is in the range of 7–19% depending upon the involved suture.

**E.** The only proven treatment is **surgery.** In positional molding (not true craniosynostosis) positioning regimens and custom helmets may be effective.

   **1.** In some cases surgery is a medical necessity to allow for normal brain growth, to prevent visual impairment, and to correct intracranial hypertension.

   **2.** Surgical procedures vary with the type of synostosis and within each category there are a variety of operative procedures in use.

   **3.** Single-suture synostosis correction should take place before 1 year of age, optimally before 4 months, to allow normal brain growth to help normalize skull shape.

   **4.** Transfusions are required in about 50% of cases, depending on the surgical technique used.

## IV. TYPES

  **A. Scaphocephaly** (sagittal synostosis)

   **1.** Synostosis affecting only the sagittal suture.

   **2.** The involved cranium is characterized by an elongated, narrow skull from front to back. The biparietal diameter is usually the narrowest part of the skull.

   **3.** Skull expansion occurs primarily at the coronal and lambdoid sutures, resulting in frontal bossing and a prominent occiput.

   **4.** Ridging along the fused sagittal suture is common.

   **5.** Also called dolichocephaly, keel-shaped head, and boat-shaped head.

   **6.** There is a strong male predominance (80%).

   **7.** There are a number of approaches to correcting this defect. Most of these are variations on the sagittal or parasagittal craniectomies that can be done with or without an interposition substance.

  **B. Trigonocephaly** (metopic synostosis)

   **1.** The metopic suture is one of the first sutures to fuse. Premature closure of this suture results in a pointed and angular forehead with a prominent midline bony ridge.

   **2.** The orbits are angled inward, causing hypotelorism.

   **3.** Of particular note, trigonocephaly is occasionally associated with intracranial abnormalities and other congenital abnormalities. A CT or MRI scan is indicated in the evaluation of these patients.

   **4.** These patients may have some degree of mental retardation.

    **5.** The surgical repair of this anomaly involves correction at the frontal base. Orbital advancement may be required to achieve a good cosmetic result.

**C. Frontal plagiocephaly** (coronal synostosis)

    **1.** Premature fusion of one coronal suture results in marked facial asymmetry. There is associated involvement of the sphenofrontal suture on the same side.

    **2.** The involved side has a flattened frontal region with the contralateral side showing a compensatory outward bulging. The nose is canted toward the affected side. The ipsilateral ear is moved forward and more inferior when compared with the uninvolved side. The affected orbit is small.

    **3.** The deformity of the skull base can cause displacement of the mandibular condyle with subsequent distortion of mandibular growth ultimately causing dental malocclusion.

    **4.** Plain radiographs show the pathognomonic **"harlequin eye"** which results from elevation of the sphenoid ridge.

    **5.** Intrauterine constraint and torticollis may also promote the development of plagiocephaly. This can be treated initially with positioning and therapy, but may ultimately require surgery.

    **6.** The surgical correction of this anomaly includes a frontal craniotomy with correction of the orbital deformity.

**D. Occipital plagiocephaly** (lambdoid synostosis)

    **1.** The premature fusion of the lambdoid suture causes flattening of the involved occipital region with prominence in the ipsilateral frontal region.

    **2.** True lambdoid synostosis is rare.

    **3.** A similar appearance is noted in infants due to postural deformation, cranio-occipital malformations, cervical spine anomalies (Klippel-Feil syndrome), and torticollis.

    **4.** Cervical spine radiographs should be performed in patients with occipital plagiocephaly who do not demonstrate fusion of the lambdoid suture.

    **5.** Multiple surgical procedures, from bilateral occipital craniectomies with reversal of the bone flaps to strip craniectomies have been described.

**E. Oxycephaly**

    **1.** Fusion of multiple cranial sutures produces a generally conical head shape which varies somewhat depending on the sutures involved.

    **2.** Also called brachycephaly (short head), acrocephaly (pointed head), and turricephaly (tower head).

    **3.** This requires surgical intervention to allow for normal brain growth and prevent visual impairment and the development of increased ICP.

**V. CRANIOFACIAL SYNDROMES.** The association of craniosynostosis with abnormalities of the facial skeleton is the basis of a group of disorders known as craniofacial syndromes or craniofacial dysmorphisms.

    **A. Crouzon's syndrome.** This autosomal dominant (variably expressed) disorder is characterized by coronal synostosis with involvement of the basal skull sutures. Facial abnormalities include maxillary hypoplasia, shallow orbits with exophthalmos, and hypertelorism with or without divergent strabismus. A conductive hearing loss is frequently seen. Hydrocephalus, mental retardation, seizures, and optic atrophy may be seen in the syndrome.

**B. Apert syndrome** (acrocephalosyndactyly). This disorder has an autosomal dominant inheritance with a large number of fresh mutations. Craniosynostosis is variable, but most commonly involves the coronal sutures. There is midfacial hypoplasia with flat facies, hypertelorism, downslanting of the palpebral fissures, and strabismus. Associated anomalies include syndactyly (osseous or cutaneous), pyloric stenosis, ectopic anus, and pulmonary aplasia.

**C. Kleeblattschädel syndrome.** An autosomal recessive, variably expressed anomaly characterized by a trilobed skull (cloverleaf skull), low-set ears, and facial deformities. It may occur as an isolated entity or associated with thanatophoric dwarfism. Hydrocephalus secondary to aqueductal stenosis may be present.

**D. Carpenter's syndrome.** An autosomal recessive disorder most commonly seen with brachycephaly, although other sutures may be involved. Lateral displacement of the inner canthi is frequently seen. Brachydactyly of the hands, syndactyly of the feet, and hypogenitalism complete the syndrome.

**E. Saethre-Chotzen syndrome.** This has an autosomal dominant inheritance with wide variance in expression. Brachycephaly with maxillary hypoplasia, a prominent ear crus, and syndactyly are the hallmarks of this disorder. Mental retardation may be seen.

**F. Pfeiffer's syndrome.** This disorder has autosomal dominant inheritance with frequent new mutations. Brachycephaly with or without involvement of the sagittal sutures is seen in association with hypertelorism, upslanting palpebral fissures, and a narrow maxilla. The thumbs and toes are notably broad. Mental retardation, Chiari malformation, and hydrocephalus are seen less frequently.

**G. Baller-Gerold syndrome.** An autosomal recessive disorder characterized by craniosynostosis, dysplastic ears, and radial aplasia and hypoplasia. Optic atrophy, conductive hearing loss, and spina bifida occulta are occasionally seen.

**H. Summitt syndrome.** An autosomal recessive disorder with craniosynostosis, variable syndactyly, and gynecomastia.

**I. Herrmann-Opitz syndrome.** An autosomal dominant disorder with variable expression characterized by craniosynostosis, brachysyndactyly, syndactyly of the hands, and absent toes.

**J. Herrmann-Pallister-Opitz syndrome.** An autosomal dominant, variably expressed syndrome involving craniosynostosis with microcrania, cleft lip and palate, symmetrically malformed limbs, and radial aplasia.

# Encephalopathies

The term encephalopathy refers to a disorder affecting the brain that results in an alteration in the level of consciousness. A variety of conditions can disrupt normal cerebral function. Some of these present primarily with encephalopathic changes and others are merely accompanied by alterations in the level of consciousness as part of the overall presentation. Encephalopathy in general, and some of its specific causes are discussed below.

## I. GENERAL
A. A wide range of disorders can cause changes in the level of consciousness and result in encephalopathy (Table 18-1).
B. Trauma, hypoxic-ischemia, and infection are the leading causes of childhood encephalopathy.
C. **Pathophysiology**
1. **Bilateral, diffuse cortical processes** (edema, encephalitis) alter global cerebral function and cause an alteration in the level of consciousness. The hallmark of global cortical impairment is the preservation of brainstem function. Metabolic and acid-base disorders often affect global cortical function.
2. **Supratentorial mass lesions** (tumor, infection, hematoma) can cause downward herniation with compression of the brainstem and impairment of the reticular activating system. Altered level of consciousness, focal neurological deficits, and progressive brainstem dysfunction suggest a mass lesion with herniation.
3. **Brainstem lesions** (tumor, vascular, infection) alter consciousness by direct impingement on the reticular activating system. Focal brainstem findings, often with intact or ipsilateral extremity findings, suggest a brainstem mass.
D. **Treatment**
1. Management of the underlying causative problem.
2. Treatment of elevated ICP (see Chapter 20).
3. Supportive care as needed. Mechanical ventilation can be both supportive and therapeutic in the management of elevated ICP.

## II. HYPOXIC-ISCHEMIC ENCEPHALOPATHY
A. Intrauterine, antepartum, intrapartum, or perinatal asphyxia often results in death. Survivors often have significant neurological impairment, including epilepsy, mental retardation, and cerebral palsy.
B. HIE of infancy has been divided into mild, moderate, and severe, based on clinical severity.
1. **Mild HIE.** Postnatal lethargy, jitteriness, sympathetic hyperactivity (pupillary dilatation, tachycardia), and head lag. Symptoms abate after the first week and complete recovery can be expected.
2. **Moderate HIE.** Lethargy and obtundation persisting for at least the first 12 hours of life. Hypotonia, jitteriness, and proximal muscle weakness are present. Some infants rap-

**Table 18-1. Causes of encephalopathy**

Hypoxic-ischemic injury
Intracranial infection
Systemic infection
Seizure disorders
Intracranial mass lesions
Intracranial vascular lesions
Trauma
Reye's syndrome
Electrolyte imbalance
Acid-base disorders
Renal failure
Hepatic failure
Metabolic disorders
Endocrine disorders

idly improve within the first 3 days of life. Others progress to further impairment in consciousness, becoming unresponsive to stimulation. Seizures may develop and are associated with a poor prognosis. Apneic spells are not uncommon.

3. **Severe HIE.** Unresponsive at birth, requiring ventilatory assistance. Seizures, profound hypotonia, absent Moro's reflex, and impaired sucking and swallowing are evident. Signs of elevated ICP (bulging fontanelle, suture separation) are associated with a poor prognosis.

C. Several characteristic neuropathological lesions result from HIE.

1. **Generalized and cortical (laminar) necrosis.** Neurons of the cerebellar and cortical cortices are affected. The Purkinje cells of the cerebellum are particularly vulnerable. Similarly, the third, fifth, and sixth cerebral cortical laminae and the depths of the sulci are most susceptible. Symmetric, selective tissue necrosis in the inferior colliculi and other brainstem nuclei is common. This pattern of damage is thought to be consistent with hypotension of slow onset but long duration. Clinically, mental retardation, cerebral palsy, and epilepsy are seen with this pattern of injury.

2. **Periventricular leukomalacia** refers to a limited pattern of tissue damage with multiple small foci of tissue necrosis centered in the periventricular white matter. This is frequently noted in infants with birth weights less than 1500 g and is thought to be related to ischemia at the periventricular arterial border. Clinically this is associated with spastic diplegia.

3. **Arterial border zone (watershed) pattern** of injury describes ischemic changes between the territories of major cerebral and cerebellar arteries. Most commonly, the parieto-occipital region is affected. The mechanism of injury is thought to be related to an abrupt fall in systemic blood pressure. The infarction is often hemorrhagic as a result of reperfusion through damaged capillaries. Clinical findings

are correlated with the region damaged by ischemia.

4. **Arterial supply territory pattern** describes necrosis within the distribution of a major cerebral vessel. **Porencephalies** develop in the affected region or regions. The term **multicystic encephalomalacia** has been used to describe multiple regions of cavitated necrosis. Fifty percent of cases involve the middle cerebral artery distribution. This pattern of ischemia is usually due to periods of significantly reduced blood flow. Clinical findings are related to the region of injury.

5. **Status marmoratus** is a pattern of neuronal loss, gliosis, and hypermyelination within the caudate, putamen, globus pallidus, and thalamus. The basal ganglia appear marbled on gross examination. Clinically this condition is characterized by mental retardation, spastic quadriparesis, choreoathetosis, and rigidity.

6. **Sommer's sector (h-1)** of the hippocampus is particularly vulnerable to hypoxia. Chronic damage to this region can result in **mesial temporal sclerosis** or **hippocampal sclerosis,** which has been associated with epilepsy.

## D. Diagnosis

1. **History.** A history consistent with potential neonatal anoxia is elicited in most cases.

2. **Examination.**

3. **EEG** is useful for determining the severity of the injury and has some prognostic value. The degree of amplitude suppression reflects the severity of the injury. In the first 24 hours, EEG demonstrates voltage suppression and slowing. Subsequently, a periodic pattern with intervals of suppression interspersed with bursts of asynchronous sharp waves develops. Sixty-four percent of patients with EEG suppression of at least 1 week's duration will have neurological impairment. All patients with suppression persisting for 2 weeks will be neurologically impaired.

4. **Radiographic investigation** (US/CT/MRI) can help distinguish the type of injury as outlined above.

5. **Treatment** involves the correction of hypoxia and acidosis. Administration of anticonvulsant agents for seizures is appropriate. Elevated ICP may require aggressive therapy (see Chapter 20).

6. **Outcome** is based on the type and severity of injury. The mortality rate with HIE is in the range of 7%. Thirty-four percent of survivors will have neurological impairment.

## III. BILIRUBIN ENCEPHALOPATHIES

### A. General

1. Bilirubin is the final catabolic product of heme, which is the primary source of circulating hemoglobin.

2. The normal turnover of red blood cells accounts for 75% of the bilirubin produced daily.

3. Bilirubin is produced in the reticuloendothelial system and transported bound to albumin to the liver, where it is converted to an excretable conjugate that is eliminated in bile.

4. Hyperbilirubinemia results when the normal metabolism

of bilirubin does not or cannot occur. Causes of hyper-bilirubinemia include disorders of conjugation, endocrine disorders, breakdown of extravascular blood, blood dyscrasias, and hemolytic anemia due to Rh or ABO incompatibility.

5. The most important determinant of central nervous system damage from bilirubin is the serum level of unconjugated bilirubin that crosses the intact and disrupted blood-brain barrier. Other predisposing factors to bilirubin encephalopathy include low birth weight, prematurity, hypoxia, acidosis, and sepsis.

6. Neurons (as opposed to glia) appear to have increased susceptibility to bilirubin injury.

7. **Neuropathology.** Patterns of bilirubin staining have been established. Selected nuclear groups, including the substantia nigra, globus pallidus, Ammon's horn, inferior olive, dentate nucleus, and the oculomotor, vestibulocochlear, facial, and hypoglossal cranial nerve nuclei are preferentially stained. A second pattern of more diffuse staining is noted in association with periventricular leukomalacia or other destructive lesions. Evidence of neuronal necrosis (pyknosis and eosinophilic degeneration) in affected regions is common.

## B. Acute bilirubin encephalopathy (kernicterus)

1. The incidence of kernicterus (nuclear jaundice) in infants of less than 32 weeks' gestation is 25%. Only 2% of term infants are affected. These numbers reflect the changing epidemiology of this condition, which was previously seen in association with hemolytic anemias and isoimmunization (Rh or ABO incompatibility). Kernicterus is now seen most commonly in low-birth-weight infants. This supports the notion that prior damage to the CNS predisposes the brain to bilirubin accumulation and damage.

2. **Features.** Lethargy, hypotonia, and poor sucking are apparent early. Subsequently, hypertonia and opisthotonos develop. Ultimately, athetosis, dystonia, impaired vertical gaze and other gaze palsies, auditory impairment, and mental retardation become evident. Tone may ultimately be increased or decreased.

3. **Diagnosis** is based on exam and a neonatal history of perinatal anoxia or prematurity. Kernicterus can develop even in children with only mild elevations of bilirubin if predisposing conditions are present.

4. **Treatment** is primarily preventive. Early detection and prevention in patients at risk (i.e., the treatment of Rh incompatibility with anti-Rh immune globulin) is essential. Careful screening and surveillance of low-birth-weight infants for levels of serum bilirubin and albumin and avoidance of hypoxia and sepsis are important. Aggressive management of hyperbilirubinemia with phototherapy and exchange transfusion should be instituted early.

5. **Outcome.** Bilirubin encephalopathy is characterized by an evolving course.

   a. Infants display hypotonia and poor feeding.

    **b.** Between 1 and 4 years of age, extrapyramidal dysfunction (athetosis, dystonia), gaze pareses (predominantly impaired vertical gaze), and auditory impairment become evident.

    **c.** Nearly 40% of afflicted children have an IQ of 90–100. One quarter of patients have an IQ less than 70.

## IV. REYE'S SYNDROME

**A.** A viral-induced systemic disorder of mitochondrial dysfunction manifested by encephalopathy and fatty infiltration of the liver and other organs.

**B.** Reye's syndrome occurs in conjunction with, or after, a viral illness. There is statistical confirmation of an increased incidence of Reye's syndrome if salicylates are administered during a viral infection. The recognition of this fact has led to a decrease in the incidence of Reye's syndrome, with only 200–500 cases now reported annually.

**C.** Infants and children of all ages are affected, with 90% of cases occurring in children under the age of 15. Rare cases have been reported in adults.

**D. Features**

    **1.** Prodromal illness with one of at least 19 viral illnesses, most commonly influenza A, influenza B, or varicella. There is no correlation between the severity of the antecedent viral illness and the severity of the encephalopathy.

    **2.** There is a predictable clinical course that Lovejoy divided into stages. The rate of progression is variable, but may be as rapid as 24 or fewer hours. Not all cases progress beyond stage III.

        **a. Stage I.** Lethargy, confusion, vomiting, and evidence of hepatic dysfunction (elevated serum transaminases, elevated serum ammonia, prolonged prothrombin time).

        **b. Stage II.** Delirium, agitation, hyperactive DTR, hyperventilation, decorticate posturing, and evidence of hepatic dysfunction.

        **c. Stage III.** Obtundation, hyperventilation, decorticate posturing, preserved oculovestibular and pupillary reflexes, evidence of hepatic dysfunction.

        **d. Stage IV.** Coma, decerebrate posturing, Cheyne-Stokes respiration, loss of pupillary and light reflexes.

        **e. Stage V.** Unresponsiveness, flaccidity, seizures, Cheyne-Stokes respiration or respiratory arrest, loss of brainstem reflexes, and fixed, dilated pupils.

    **3.** Fever, hepatomegaly, and absence of jaundice.

**E. Diagnosis**

    **1.** History and examination. Often the antecedent viral illness is mild and not appreciated unless inquired about specifically.

    **2.** Elevated serum transaminases (SGOT, SGPT).

    **3.** Hypoglycemia.

    **4.** Hyperammonemia.

    **5.** Prothrombin time is initially prolonged, but returns to normal within several days.

    **6.** EEG is consistent with a diffuse encephalopathy.

    **7.** Free fatty acidemia and mild organic and amino acidemias are often noted.

8. **Liver biopsy** is definitive with histopathology by light and electron microscopy demonstrating microvesicular steatosis, glycogen depletion, intracellular lipid droplets, mitochondrial abnormalities, proliferating peroxisomes, and empty Golgi membranes.

9. Differential diagnosis includes encephalopathy due to viral hepatitis (distinguished by liver biopsy), valproic acid hepatotoxicity, systemic carnitine deficiency, and ornithine deficiency.

F. **Course.** The course is variable, with some cases being mild and self-limited, and others progressing rapidly to death.

**Table 18-2. Metabolic causes of encephalopathy**

**Hypernatremia**
Inadequate water intake
Salt loading
Excessive water loss (diarrhea)
Hyperaldosteronism
Cushing's syndrome
Excessive evaporation (fever)

**Hyponatremia**
SIADH
Congestive heart failure
Inadequate sodium intake
Cystic fibrosis
Iatrogenic volume expansion

**Acidosis**
Hypoaldosteronism
Renal tubular acidosis
Ureteral diversions
Chronic renal failure
Diabetic ketoacidosis
Lactic acidosis
Inadequate pulmonary excretion of $CO_2$ (asthma, neuromuscular disorders, brain injury)

**Alkalosis**
Hyperventilation
Pulmonary embolism
HCl loss (renal GI)

**Hypoglycemia**
Insulin administration with diabetes mellitus

**Hypochloremia**

**Hypocalcemia and hypomagnesemia**
Hypoparathyroidism
Pseudohypoparathyroidism
Vitamin D deficiency

**Hypercalcemia**
Hyperparathyroidism
Williams syndrome (hypercalcemia, elfin facies syndrome)

**G. Treatment**
   **1. Stage I and II** can usually be treated with intravenous hypertonic glucose, insulin, and management of electrolyte disturbances. Patients should be kept euvolemic and overhydration in particular should be avoided.
   **2.** Bleeding diathesis should be corrected as needed with fresh frozen plasma and vitamin K.
   **3.** Control of increased ICP should be aggressive, because ICP is often the cause of significant morbidity and mortality (see Chapter 20).
**H. Outcome** is directly related to the severity of the disorder. Even with aggressive management the mortality rate is significant (45% of stage III, 65% of stage IV, and nearly 100% of stage V).

## V. METABOLIC ENCEPHALOPATHY
**A.** Normal cerebral function can be impaired by a variety of metabolic abnormalities (Table 18-2).
**B. Features**
   **1.** Altered level of consciousness manifested by irritability, lethargy, or decreased general alertness.
   **2.** Change in respiratory pattern with hyperventilation, Cheyne-Stokes respiration, or apneic spells.
   **3.** Seizures.
   **4.** Decorticate or decerebrate posturing can develop.
**C. Diagnosis** is by history and exam. Other causes of encephalopathy must be considered.
**D. Treatment** involves correction of the underlying disorder.
**E. Outcome** is based on the duration of symptoms prior to correction and the degree of impairment at the time of intervention.

## VI. HEPATIC ENCEPHALOPATHY
**A.** Liver damage by acute or chronic conditions may result in neurological sequelae. In children, the most common causes of hepatic encephalopathy are acute infectious hepatitis, and drug and toxin ingestion (acetaminophen, valproic acid, poisonous mushrooms).
**B.** The CNS symptoms are thought to be related to elevated levels of serum ammonia.
**C. Features**
   **1.** Altered level of consciousness.
   **2.** Asterixis.
   **3.** Respiratory changes (hyperventilation, Cheyne-Stokes respiration).
   **4.** Chorea.
   **5.** Coagulopathy with risk of intracranial hemorrhage.
**D. Diagnosis** of the underlying liver disorder aids the diagnosis of hepatic encephalopathy.
**E. Treatment** is supportive. Management of hypoglycemia, coagulopathy, renal failure, and electrolyte disturbance predominates. Nutrition should be provided with minimal protein and supplemental branched-chain amino acids. Liver transplant for chronic hepatic failure is an option.
**F. Outcome** is based on the severity of the liver disorder.

## VII. OTHER ENCEPHALOPATHIES
**A. Toxic.** The intentional or accidental ingestion of prescrip-

tion drugs or poisons may cause encephalopathy. These are most common in 1- to 4-year-olds. Older children may develop encephalopathy from substance abuse.

**B. Burns.** Five percent of children with burns on over 30% of their body surface area develop an encephalopathy that is probably related to the multiple metabolic abnormalities associated with severe burns.

# Head Trauma

Head trauma is the third leading cause of death in children less than 1 year of age, and the leading cause of death in children over 1 year of age. It is responsible for significant morbidity and mortality in the pediatric age group. The assessment and management of head trauma are discussed in this chapter. Unique features of pediatric head trauma are also addressed.

## I. GENERAL
A. For ages 0–4 years the incidence of head injury is 150:100,000. This increases to 550:100,000 for ages 15–24.
B. Males sustain 2 times as many head injuries as females, and are 4 times more likely to have a fatal head injury.
C. Causes of head trauma include falls, motor vehicle accidents, flying missiles, child abuse, and birth.

## II. INITIAL ASSESSMENT
A. As with any trauma patient, the ABCs must be given first priority. Often head injury occurs in the setting of multiple trauma. In these cases, the patient should also be evaluated by a general surgeon and other consultants as needed to ensure optimal medical care.
   1. Extension of the neck to establish an airway should be avoided prior to radiographic evaluation of the cervical spine. An airway can be established **without** extension of the neck.
   2. Hypovolemic shock is usually not caused by intracranial hemorrhage except in small infants. However, scalp lacerations and skull fractures into a sinus may cause hypovolemia.
   3. High cervical injuries can cause hypovolemia through the mechanism of spinal shock and the loss of sympathetic tone. This should be treated initially with volume and then dopamine as needed. Refer to Chapter 21 for further detail.

## III. NEUROLOGICAL EXAMINATION
A. **History** obtained from the patient, if conscious, or witnesses and EMS regarding loss of consciousness, mechanism of injury, and evolution of the neurological examination is imperative. A good history provides important diagnostic information and guides the examination process. Amnesia is indicative of a loss of consciousness.
B. **Mechanism of injury**
   1. Maximal primary neurological injury occurs at the time of impact.
   2. Penetrating injury directly disrupts tissue and can cause mass effect through creation of a clot or introduction of a foreign body.
   3. Hypotension and hypoxia both contribute to nervous system damage.
   4. At a cellular level, alterations in neurotransmitters and calcium homeostasis may explain some of the changes that are seen.
C. **Severity of injury**
   1. **Mild injury.** Crying, vomiting, pallor, and apathy are

117

noted in cases of mild injury. The majority of these children recover in 24 to 48 hours without sequelae. **Pediatric concussion syndrome** refers to a relatively minor trauma to the head with development of nausea, vomiting, lethargy, and pallor delayed by hours. Children usually return to normal within 24 hours.

   **2.Major injury** (see below).

**D. Coma scale**

   **1.**In the description of head injury, terms such as comatose and obtunded are not useful. Rather, a description of the patient's response to the environment, as well as the level of consciousness, pupillary responses, and motor and reflex responses should be detailed.

   **2.Glasgow coma scale.** (Table 19-1).

   **3.**Because infants and children are not able to perform to command, and do not necessarily have the ability to speak conversationally, a modified pediatric coma scale should be used. (Table 19-2).

**E. Unconscious patients**

   **1.**Brainstem function should be assessed in the unconscious patient to establish the level of the lesion. This should include pupillary response, caloric response, respiratory patterns, and movement.

     **a. Diencephalon**

       **(1)** Conjugate tonic eye deviation in response to cold-water caloric tests.

       **(2)** Pupils are small and reactive to light.

       **(3)** Purposeful or decorticate posturing.

       **(4)** Cheyne-Stokes respiration.

     **b. Midbrain**

Table 19-1. Glasgow coma scale

|  |  | Score |
| --- | --- | --- |
| **Eye opening** | Spontaneous | 4 |
|  | To command | 3 |
|  | To pain | 2 |
|  | No response | 1 |
| **Best motor** | Obeys | 6 |
|  | Localizes | 5 |
|  | Withdrawal | 4 |
|  | Flexor | 3 |
|  | Extensor | 2 |
|  | No response | 1 |
| **Best verbal** | Oriented and conversant | 5 |
|  | Disoriented and conversant | 4 |
|  | Inappropriate words | 3 |
|  | Unclear | 2 |
|  | No response | 1 |

Table 19-2. Pediatric coma scale

|  |  | Score |
| --- | --- | --- |
| **Eye opening** | Spontaneous | 4 |
|  | To voice | 3 |
|  | To pain | 2 |
|  | No response | 1 |
| **Best motor** | Flexes/extends | 4 |
|  | Withdraws | 3 |
|  | Hypertonic | 2 |
|  | Flaccid | 1 |
| **Best verbal** | Cries | 3 |
|  | Spontaneous respiration | 2 |
|  | Apneic | 1 |

      (1) Dysconjugate eye deviation in response to cold-water caloric tests.

      (2) Midposition, nonreactive pupils.

      (3) Decerebrate posturing.

      (4) Hyperventilation.

   c. **Pons**

      (1) No response to caloric stimulation with cold-water caloric testing.

      (2) Pinpoint pupils, reactive to light.

      (3) Flaccidity.

      (4) Apneustic breathing.

  **2.** Prior to the instillation of cold water into the ear canal, otoscopic examination should be performed to assess the integrity of the tympanic membrane. If the tympanic membrane is not intact, caloric tests should not be performed.

 **F. Radiographic examination.** Once stabilized, appropriate neurodiagnostic studies should be obtained.

  **1. AP and lateral c-spines** to rule out any obvious cervical trauma. These films are important should the patient require operative intervention where manipulation of the neck for positioning is required. Further views (oblique, flexion, extension) should be obtained as indicated.

  **2. Brain CT without contrast.**

  **3. Thoracic and lumbosacral spine** films as indicated.

 **G.** The radiographic studies and clinical exam together place the patient in an operative or nonoperative category. Monitoring and management of ICP are discussed in Chapter 20.

**IV. OPERATIVE LESIONS**

 **A. Scalp lacerations.** Clean thoroughly, debride as necessary, and close primarily.

 **B. Skull fractures** requiring operative intervention include the following.

  **1.** Fractures that are depressed more than 1 cm and are located between the coronal and lambdoid sutures. This general principle is based on the fact that these fractures are more likely to be associated with cerebral lacerations, and hence posttraumatic epilepsy. There is some flexibility regarding this rule, and the location of the fracture, condition of the patient, and depth of the depression should all be taken into account when making the decision to operate. Depressed fractures overlying the sagittal sinus, transverse sinus, or torcula may be best managed nonoperatively. Those over the forehead may need to be elevated.

2. **Open comminuted depressed fractures** are fractures that are exposed through a scalp laceration. These cases need to be operatively debrided and sutured to prevent osteomyelitis, cerebritis, and other complications. Open linear skull fractures and small step-off fractures can be treated with thorough cleaning and debriding followed by primary closure in the emergency room.

3. **Fractures overlying vascular channels** such as the middle meningeal groove should raise concern for the possibility of an epidural hematoma. They need not be surgically explored if no underlying bleeding is found on CT examination.

4. **Diastatic fractures** (see below)

## C. Epidural hematomas

1. Can be arterial or venous in origin.

2. They are often associated with trauma to the temporal region that causes disruption of the middle meningeal artery.

3. In children they often occur without a fracture.

4. The classical presentation with a **lucid interval** occurs in only 10% of patients, and even less often in the pediatric population.

5. CT examination shows a lens-shaped collection of blood.

6. **Management**

   a. Minimal epidural hematomas may be treated conservatively. However, it must be recognized that the patient is at risk to decline, and appropriate observation and intervention are essential.

   b. Significant lesions should be surgically evacuated. Venous epidural hematomas are generally associated with a more prolonged course. In patients with minor trauma who do not improve within 24–48 hours, a CT scan should be obtained or repeated to rule out the development of an epidural hematoma.

## D. Subdural hematomas

1. Subdural hematomas are different in infants than in older children. In infants they are frequently associated with child abuse.

2. They may present **acutely** with increased ICP and retinal hemorrhages, or **subacutely** with new bleeding into a chronic subdural hematoma. **Chronic** cases can develop macrocephaly and, ultimately, signs of increased ICP.

3. **Treatment**

   a. In infants these lesions can be approached by medically controlling the increased ICP in combination with external subdural drainage.

**b.** An acute lesion that causes sufficient mass effect in an older child should be approached surgically.

**c.** More chronic lesions may require subdural to peritoneal shunting.

**d.** Craniotomies with membrane stripping are of historical interest only.

**E. Traumatic intracerebral hemorrhage** usually occurs as small white-matter hemorrhages. If a substantial clot occurs, which is unusual, it should be removed surgically. Intracerebral hemorrhage related to birth injury is covered in Chapter 7.

**F. Gunshot wounds**

1. Gunshot wounds to the head should be approached surgically when survival is feasible. Debridement of the wound with removal of devitalized brain and bone, as well as bullet fragments where possible, should be accomplished. The dura mater should be repaired.

2. Copper-jacketed missiles have been reported to migrate intracranially. This should be considered in the surgical approach.

3. **BBs and air pellets** can perforate the cranium in children. The same principles as for gunshot wounds apply; however, the entrance wound is often small and requires no operative therapy. If the pellet is deep or crosses the midline it can be left in place. There is no increased incidence of delayed brain abscess when BBs are left in place. A 10-day course of intravenous ampicillin and gentamycin should be given if a nonoperative approach is taken.

**G. Penetrating injuries.** The region of the medial canthus is particularly prone to penetrating injuries. The penetrating object may extend intracranially and these injuries can result in extensive neurological damage, including hemiparesis and endocrine abnormalities.

**V. NONOPERATIVE TRAUMA**

**A. Skull fractures**

1. **Linear skull fractures**

   **a.** Should be distinguished from vascular markings and sutures. In general, linear fractures will be straighter than vascular channels and go in a different direction than vascular markings seen on x-ray.

   **b.** Linear fractures may extend from suture to suture, buttress to buttress, or buttress to suture.

   **c.** Fractures that cross the suture line are more significant because they involve more force and can cause dural tears.

2. **Diastatic fractures**

   **a.** Occur as either split sutures or widened fractures.

   **b.** Commonly occur in children because the sutures are not completely fused. They may separate, return to position, and go undetected.

   **c.** On x-ray examination one table of the bone may appear elevated, depending on the tangent.

   **d.** These usually resolve without intervention. If the underlying dura mater has been damaged, complications such as a growing fracture (**leptomeningeal cyst**) may become evident at follow-up.

**3. Basal skull fractures**

  **a.** Basal fractures are difficult to see on plain x-ray, and are better visualized on CT.

  **b.** They may be clinically diagnosed by the presence of a Battle's sign, raccoon's eye, or CSF leak.

  **c.** Patients who sustain fractures extending through the carotid canal may warrant further investigation with arteriography.

  **d.** Longitudinal fractures through the temporal bone may disrupt the tympanic membrane or auditory ossicles, or cause injury to the facial nerve.

  **e.** Fractures through the occipital squamosa and extending into the foramen magnum may disrupt the petrous pyramid with injury to the cochlear-vestibular system and facial nerve.

  **f.** Basal skull fractures can cause CSF otorrhea or rhinorrhea.

   **(1)** This should be treated initially with elevation of the head and observation for the development of meningitis.

   **(2)** There is controversy about the use of prophylactic antibiotics. In children, antibiotics should be used in particular if there is a history of recent or recurrent ear infection.

   **(3)** The vast majority of leaks will seal within 48 hours. Leaks persisting beyond 1 week require further investigation and treatment.

**B. Concussion**

  **1.** Concussion refers to a transitory alteration in neurological function caused by a blow to the head.

  **2.** Patients with a brief concussion should be observed closely for 24–48 hours by a responsible individual.

  **3.** Longer concussions should be observed in the hospital and may require longer observation.

**C. Contusions**

  **1.** Contusions are the result of trauma to the head sufficient to cause an identifiable lesion such as a hemorrhage on CT scan.

  **2.** These patients should be observed in the hospital for 48–72 hours to ensure that further compromise does not occur with brain swelling.

  **3.** Swelling reaches a peak at 48–72 hours after the injury.

**D. Diffuse axonal injury** is a term that suggests injury sustained with angular deceleration. There is extensive damage to axons within the white matter, documented by shear hemorrhages on CT.

**E. ICP monitoring** should be instituted in patients with a coma scale less than 5. Patients with a shift on CT scan and a coma scale of 6–8 should also be managed with ICP monitoring. The management of ICP is discussed in Chapter 20.

## VI. HERNIATION SYNDROMES

**A. Central transtentorial herniation** occurs as a result of diffuse cerebral edema or a central supratentorial mass lesion. As the brainstem is displaced caudally, a clinical rostrocaudal deterioration occurs.

1. Change in mental status.
2. Small, reactive pupils progressing to midposition unreactive pupils.
3. Cheyne-Stokes respiration.
4. Decorticate posturing progressing to decerebrate posturing.
5. May progress to death.

**B. Uncal herniation** occurs when a lateral mass effect causes the uncus to herniate over the edge of the tentorium.

1. With or without change in mental status.
2. Pupillary dilatation ipsilateral to the mass.
3. Ipsilateral third nerve palsy.
4. Progression to loss of consciousness.
5. Progressive loss of midbrain function.
6. Development of decerebration and hyperventilation.
7. Death.

**C. Subfalcine herniation** refers to herniation of the cingulate gyrus under the falx cerebri as a result of a lateral mass effect. This may compromise circulation in the ipsilateral anterior cerebral artery. A contralateral loculated ventricle may develop as CSF outflow through the foramen of Monro becomes obstructed.

**D. Tonsillar herniation** involves herniation of the cerebellar tonsils through the foramen magnum as a result of a mass lesion within the posterior fossa. This is most often manifested by a compromise in respiration through its compressive effect on the medulla.

**E. Upward herniation** may occur with increased pressure in the infratentorial compartment, such as with a medulloblastoma. This may be precipitated by decompression of the supratentorial compartment with ventricular drainage. Acutely, the result is a loss of consciousness and impaired upward gaze.

## VII. UNIQUE FEATURES OF PEDIATRIC HEAD TRAUMA

**A. Flash edema** may occur in children even after relatively minor head injury. It is presumed to be a phenomenon of vascular engorgement associated with a loss of autoregulation. More recently this phenomenon has been renamed **cerebral hyperemia**.

**B. Growing fractures or leptomeningeal cysts** occur following a fracture in an infant or child that results in an outpouching of arachnoid through a laceration in the dura mater. With the normal pulsations of the brain there is erosion of the dura mater and bone. These typically present as a posttraumatic scalp mass.

**C. Transient blindness** occurs in some children after head injury. This usually lasts minutes to hours and resolves without sequelae. It may represent a posttraumatic migraine phenomenon.

D. **Cerebral dissolution** may occur in young children with severe brain injury. In these patients, there is preservation of the brainstem and diencephalon.

E. **Hydrocephalus** has been reported to develop in 29–72% of severe pediatric head injuries.

F. **Cephalohematoma** is seen often in infants. This is characterized by a subperiosteal collection of blood; they therefore respect the suture lines. Cephalohematomas may actually increase in size as the blood breaks down in the first week. These will resolve on their own and do not require intervention. The periosteal reaction around the resolving hematoma may create the false clinical impression of a depressed skull fracture.

G. **Seizures.** Immediate posttraumatic seizures are common in children and may make the neurological status appear worse than it really is.

## VIII. SEQUELAE

A. **Posttraumatic seizures**

1. Late seizures occur more frequently in adults than in children. However, early seizures and posttraumatic status epilepticus (usually focal) are more common in children than in adults.

2. Posttraumatic amnesia lasting beyond 24 hours, subdural hematomas, and depressed skull fractures lacerating the dura mater are all associated with an increased incidence of posttraumatic epilepsy. These factors should be considered prior to the initiation of anticonvulsant therapy.

B. **Posttraumatic migraines** occur in some children. Treatment with cyproheptadine hydrochloride is often effective.

## IX. PROGNOSIS

A. **Outcome** is based on a combination of the initial coma score, area and extent of brain damage, level of ICP, and the child's premorbid potential.

B. The mortality rate varies with the type of injury. Acute subdural hematomas have the highest mortality rate (83%) and depressed skull fractures with a cortical laceration have a mortality rate of less than 2%. The overall mortality rate for children with head injury is between 9 and 38%.

C. Ninety percent of children under the age of 15 who survive head trauma will recover to at least a moderately disabled status within 3 years.

D. Twenty percent of children with Glasgow coma scores of 5–7 will have a persistent neurological deficit. Fifty percent of children with scores of 3–4 will have a persistent neurological deficit.

E. Coma of less than 24 hours' duration rarely has obvious permanent neurological sequelae.

# Management of Increased Intracranial Pressure

Increased ICP can develop in a variety of settings. The causes and management of elevated ICP are reviewed in this chapter.

## I. INCREASED ICP
### A. Causes
1. **Trauma.** Increased ICP associated with trauma can be due to the development of a hematoma or cerebral edema. In children, the phenomenon of flash edema can occur even with apparent minor head injury (see Chapter 19).
2. **Neoplasms** often cause increased ICP through obstruction of the normal CSF pathways or through mass effect.
3. **Reye's syndrome** is associated with viral infections and concomitant salicylate use. Increased ICP is common and the effective management of increased ICP is often the single most important factor in outcome. This condition is discussed in greater detail in Chapter 18.
4. **Encephalopathies** (see Chapter 18).
5. **Congenital conditions** such as **hydrocephalus** and **Dandy-Walker syndrome.**

### B. Pathophysiology
1. The **Monro-Kellie doctrine** states that in the enclosed craniospinal axis (after suture and fontanelle closure), brain, CSF, and blood represent incompressible components. If a change in volume occurs in one of these components, such as an increase in CSF with hydrocephalus, either a reciprocal change occurs with one of the other components or an increase in pressure will occur. If a new component is added, such as a neoplasm, one of the three normal compartments must compensate, or elevated pressure will develop.
2. The pressure-volume curve (Figure 20-1) is nearly horizontal until the compensatory capacity of the blood, brain, and CSF is exhausted. At this point, the curve becomes steeper, as the compliance of the system has been exhausted, and small increases in volume lead to large increases in pressure. A thorough understanding of this curve is essential for the effective management of increased ICP.
3. Raised ICP in the infant is unique because of the compliance of the skull prior to suture closure. While compliance of the skull can temporize the effects of increased ICP in the chronic setting, it is of little benefit in the setting of acutely increased ICP. In infants and young children, it is important to remember that one is dealing with an immature nervous system that is continuing to develop.

## II. DIAGNOSIS
A. In the acute setting increased ICP is associated with a poor neurological examination. The Glasgow coma score is likely to be less than 7. The **Cushing response** of hypertension,

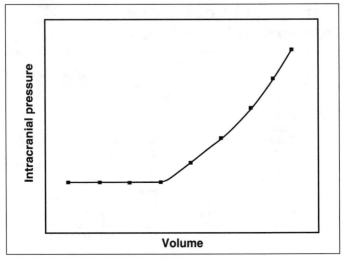

**Fig. 20-1. Pressure-volume curve for ICP.**

bradycardia, and respiratory irregularities heralds the rapid
onset of increased ICP. In adults the Cushing response often
occurs just prior to herniation. In children it occurs sooner
and intervention can be effective in preventing herniation.

**B.** In the more chronic setting a history and physical examination will reveal one or more of the following.

   1. History of headache, often worse in the morning.
   2. Vomiting.
   3. Lethargy.
   4. Intellectual decline.
   5. Bulging fontanelle with loss of pulsations.
   6. Split sutures.
   7. Head circumference crossing percentiles.
   8. Papilledema.
   9. Parinaud's syndrome.
   10. Sixth nerve palsy.
   11. Cortical markings on x-ray.

**C. Pseudotumor cerebri (benign intracranial hyperten-
   sion)**

   1. The elevation of ICP without ventricular enlargement or
      focal neurological or radiological abnormalities.
   2. In asthmatic children this can occur as they are withdrawn
      from steroids, or after otitis media or sinusitis.
   3. **Diagnosis.** It is primarily a diagnosis of exclusion.
   4. The major concern is the risk of optic atrophy and impaired
      vision. Treatment may include furosemide, periodic lumbar
      punctures, lumboperitoneal shunting, or subtemporal
      craniectomy.

**III. MANAGEMENT**

   **A.** Mass lesions associated with trauma that are amenable to surgical treatment should be approached in this manner. Neoplasms should be treated in a similar fashion.

**B.** Hydrocephalus should be managed with spinal fluid diversion.

**C.** Increased ICP in other settings can be managed as follows.

**1.Positioning.** The patient should be kept with the head of the bed at 30–45$^0$, with the neck extended to discourage venous obstruction.

**2.Intubation and hyperventilation** to a $PCO_2$ of 25 initially. Hyperventilation provides the most rapid and effective means of lowering ICP and should be instituted early. Respiratory care in a patient with increased ICP should be meticulous. Bagged hyperventilation with 100% $O_2$ prior to frequent suctioning is important.

**3.Mannitol** is the most effective osmotic diuretic available. The initial dose is 0.25–1.00 g/kg intravenously.

**4.**The placement of a **ventriculostomy** for the management of increased ICP is preferred, since this method allows for the accurate measurement of ICP and for drainage of CSF to control ICP. **Epidural or subdural bolts and intraparenchymal catheters** can be placed to monitor pressure and guide therapy, but they do not allow for CSF drainage. Accurate measurement of ICP alone is obtained **only** if the transducer is in line to the monitor, not to the drain and monitor simultaneously.

**5.**If ICP remains elevated, one or more of the following measures can be instituted.

**a. Mannitol** can be administered at 0.25 g/kg IV q3–4 h. Sometimes mannitol may be contraindicated, as in heart failure (which may occur in very small infants), and when serum Na is > 150 or serum osmolality is > 310.

**b. Paralysis** using pancuronium (0.1 mg/kg IV) or norcuronium (0.1 mg/kg IV) as needed (only in intubated patients).

**c. Furosemide** as a drip containing D5 1/2NS with 5–10 mg furosemide/500 cc, 30 mEq KCl, and 5 mEq Na $HCO_3$/ 500 cc. This should run at two-thirds maintenance. The other one-third maintenance should be administered as Plasmanate. Furosemide can also be given as a bolus.

**6.**If ICP remains elevated, extreme measures include the use of **thiopental.**

**a.** This can be given on a prn basis (3–5 mg/kg IV) or as a continuous infusion.

**b.** Alternatively, thiopental coma can be initiated with a drip of 1–2 mg/kg/h, titrated to provide burst suppression on EEG (provided hypotension and cardiac irregularities do not occur).

**c.** It is important that the patient treated with thiopental not be hypovolemic. Patients who require this measure need very intensive monitoring.

**7.**Steroids have no demonstrated beneficial effect in the setting of head trauma. They do have a beneficial effect in the setting of edema related to brain tumors.

# Spinal Cord Injury

One to ten percent of all spine injuries occur in the pediatric population (birth to 16 years of age), making these relatively uncommon injuries. Fifty percent of these injuries occur in 15- and 16-year-olds. The vast majority is in the cervical region. Thoracolumbar injuries occur infrequently. Unique features of the pediatric spine and the management of SCI are reviewed in this chapter.

## I. GENERAL
A. Pediatric vertebral column injuries are unique. Both the type of injury sustained and the management of pediatric spinal column injuries are different because of the physical and biomechanical differences in the developing spine.
1. Immature cervical and paraspinous musculature.
2. Laxity of major ligamentous structures.
3. Horizontally oriented articular facets.
4. Wedge-shaped, incompletely ossified vertebrae.
B. The most common cause of pediatric spinal column injuries is falls. Other causes include sports, diving, MVAs, and pedestrian-related MVAs.
C. Ten to twenty percent of pediatric spine injuries involve more than one vertebral level.

## II. SCIWORA (spinal cord injury without radiographic abnormality)
A. As the name suggests, SCIWORA indicates spinal cord dysfunction without radiographic abnormalities.
B. Most commonly seen in children.
C. Comprises 15–70% of pediatric cases of SCI.
D. Presumed etiologies: transient subluxation, disruption of vascular supply, reversible disc protrusion.
E. Nearly half of reported cases have a delayed onset of symptoms.

## III. ACUTE MANAGEMENT OF SCI
A. ABCs
1. Regardless of the type of injury, the ABCs must be addressed first.
2. Cervical cord lesions result in paralysis of the intercostal musculature, which accounts for 60% of effective ventilation.
3. Cervical spine-injured patients need constant assessment for hypoventilation. A lesion above C4 also impairs diaphragmatic breathing. Unless artificial ventilation is initiated immediately, the patient will die of respiratory failure. This is a significant ethical dilemma.
B. **Immobilization.** Use of a cervical collar or stabilizing bolsters to prevent further injury. The patient should be moved as a unit.
C. **Survey.** The patient should be assessed for other injuries. In patients with a cervical or thoracic level of injury, thoracic, abdominal, and lower extremity trauma may be present without complaint of pain because of spinal cord disruption.

**D. Level.** Establish the level of injury. Priapism (unopposed parasympathetic activity) **suggests** a complete cervical lesion.

**E. Spinal shock**

1. Paralytic vasodilatation from loss of sympathetic tone below the level of the lesion.

2. Manifested by bradycardia and hypotension.

3. **Treatment** includes initial hydration to fill the dilated vascular bed, followed by dopamine, if needed, to improve vascular tone. Unless hypovolemia is clearly due to blood loss, spinal shock should be suspected. Correction of hypovolemia due to spinal shock with fluids alone can result in pulmonary edema.

4. **Duration** of spinal shock is hours to days. It may take 3–4 weeks for reflex activity to resume.

5. An intact bulbocavernosus reflex suggests the end of spinal shock.

**F. Steroids.** Currently, evidence supports the use of high-dose steroids in cases of spinal cord injury. Steroids should be instituted within 8 hours of injury or not at all. A loading dose of methylprednisolone of 30 mg/kg IV infused over 15 minutes is administered. After a 45-minute delay, a continuous infusion of methylprednisolone at a rate of 5.4 mg/kg/h is given for a total of 23 hours. Ranitidine or another $H_2$-blocker should be used in conjunction with steroid therapy. There is no reported increase in the incidence of infection or GI hemorrhage associated with this protocol.

**G. Thermoregulation.** The ability to maintain normal body temperature is impaired. Autonomic dysfunction leads to an inability to vasoconstrict or shiver to increase body temperature, or to vasodilate and sweat to decrease body temperature. In effect, the quadriplegic is a poikilotherm. Body temperature must be kept normal through artificial means.

**H. Pressure sores.** Decubiti can develop rapidly. The patient must be transferred to a soft surface as soon as possible. Histological ischemic changes are seen within 30 minutes of continuous pressure.

**I.** A **nasogastric tube** should be placed immediately to avoid aspiration and gastric distention.

**IV. RADIOGRAPHIC EVALUATION**

**A. Plain x-rays** of the spine (cervical, thoracic, lumbosacral). Normal variations in children must be considered.

1. **Pseudosubluxation.** Physiologic anterior displacement of C2 (on C3) or C3 (on C4) in children 8 and under.

2. **Enlarged predental space** (C1–odontoid process) up to 3–5 mm.

3. The dens is separated from the lateral masses by the neurocentral synchondroses and from the centrum by the subchondral synchondrosis. This may simulate a fracture on lateral c-spines until adolescence.

**B. Flexion-extension cervical spine** (should only be performed if other views are normal). Again, children have some normal variations.

1. Overriding of the anterior arch of C1 on the odontoid during

extension.
  **2.** Variable angulation between adjacent vertebrae during flexion.
**C. CT** is particularly useful in defining subtle injuries and upper cervical injuries. Sagittal reconstructions provide further information about alignment. Hemorrhage within the canal can also be delineated with CT.
**D. MRI** is not useful in defining the bony abnormalities, but provides the best imaging of the cord for evidence of contusion, disruption, or hemorrhage.

# V. LONG-TERM MANAGEMENT OF SCI

## A. Respiratory
  **1.** Intubation may be required initially. Permanent mechanical ventilation may be necessary for high cervical injuries, and this poses an ethical dilemma. Patients with cervical lesions below C4 can ultimately be trained to use diaphragmatic breathing techniques with reasonably good success.
  **2.** The cough reflex is often impaired. Aggressive pulmonary toilet (suctioning, physiotherapy, postural drainage) is essential to prevent pneumonia.

## B. Gastrointestinal
  **1. Paralytic ileus** is common. Treatment involves placement of an NG for intermittent low-wall suction with replacement of fluid, KCl, and HCL as needed. Onset may be delayed 24–48 hours, but may last weeks. Metoclopramide hydrochloride can be helpful.
  **2. Gastric/peptic ulcers** develop related to stress. Prophylactic $H_2$-blocker and sucralfate should be initiated early.
  **3. Nutrition.** As soon as possible, nutritional support should be provided. If the gut is not acceptable, then total parenteral nutrition should be started.
  **4.** A bowel program to include stool softeners and suppositories or stimulation.

## C. Neurogenic bladder
  **1.** Initially, an indwelling catheter can be placed. Acutely, a full bladder should not be emptied entirely or a vagal episode can follow with bradycardia and even cardiac arrest.
  **2.** Intermittent catheterization is effective for long-term management.

## D. Decubiti
  **1. Prophylaxis.** Frequent positioning, cleaning, vigilant nursing care, air mattresses, or rotational beds.
  **2. Treatment.** No pressure, frequent cleaning, and attention to nutrition should heal most decubiti.
  **3. Surgery** may be required for pressure sores that extend into the muscle or bone, if they are large, or not healing well. Surgery should be a last resort.

## E. Spasticity
  **1.** With a loss of cortical inhibitory impulses there is excessive, unopposed reflex activity below the level of the lesion, causing hyperreflexia, spasticity, and clonus. The primary concern with spasticity is the development of contractures.
  **2.** Aggressive physical therapy helps minimize spasticity and

its effects.

3. Drugs (baclofen, dantrolene sodium, diazepam) can be useful adjuncts.

4. **Surgical treatment** (rhizotomy, myelotomy) should be a last resort.

F. **Surgery.** Surgical intervention is rarely required in pediatric spine injuries. Immobilization however, is often required. It can be obtained with halo jacket, Minerva jacket, or skeletal traction.

G. **Rehabilitation** in an SCI center helps maximize recovery. As soon as the patient is medically stable, incorporation into a rehabilitation unit should be aggressively sought.

VI. **ASSOCIATED CONDITIONS.** Because SCI in children is uncommon, associated conditions should be considered when it occurs. A number of conditions are associated with hypermobility in the cervical region and may increase the likelihood of injury with trauma.

A. **Congenital anomalies of the odontoid** from aplasia (complete absence) to os odontoidium (apical segment separated from the base).

B. **Down syndrome**

C. **Klippel-Feil syndrome** (congenital fusion of cervical vertebrae).

D. **Morquio syndrome**

E. **Neurofibromatosis**

F. **Osteogenesis imperfecta**

G. **Spondyloepiphyseal dysplasia**

1. **SED congenita.** A dominantly transmitted condition of short-trunked dwarfism. One third of these children have neurologically compromising odontoid hypoplasia.

2. **SED tarda.** A sex-linked, recessive condition that affects the spine.

H. **Rheumatoid (childhood) arthritis** is associated with a number of cervical spine abnormalities. Subluxations (often atlantoaxial) and an "apple-core" odontoid (from erosion) occur.

# Peripheral Neuropathies

A wide variety of neuropathies develop in childhood. They may occur as isolated entities involving only the nervous system, or as part of a systemic process. Motor, sensory, or autonomic nerve fibers can be preferentially involved. Patterns of involvement aid in the diagnosis. Etiologies of neuropathies include hereditary processes, inflammation, autoimmune processes, and toxic exposures. Neuropathies with genetic transmission are important to identify so that appropriate genetic counseling can be provided to affected families.

## I. EVALUATION AND WORKUP
### A. History x
1. **Gestation.** A history of change in fetal movements during the pregnancy or compared to other pregnancies.
2. It is important to recognize that sensory symptoms may not be described by infants or very young children.
3. History of similar complaints in the extended family.
4. Potential toxin exposures at home, school, or in the environment.
5. Progression and tempo of change throughout development. Prolonged feeding times in infancy and achievement or loss of motor milestones help to define the course of the illness.

### B. Physical examination
1. In addition to the examination of the patient, examination of parents, siblings, and other family members may be indicated.
2. Patterns of involvement. In general, neuropathies have a predominantly distal effect (as compared with myopathies which have a more proximal effect). The lower extremities are typically more involved than the upper extremities. Notable exceptions to this include porphyria, GBS, CIDP, and Dejerine-Sottas disease, all of which can have more pronounced proximal weakness.
3. Motor/sensory involvement
   a. **Predominantly motor impairment.** GBS, porphyria, diphtheria, lead poisoning, HMSN-I, and HMSN-III.
   b. **Predominantly sensory impairment.** Diabetes, HSAN, leprosy, metabolic disorders, or disorders due to nutritional deficiencies.

### C. Initial workup.
Complete blood count, electrolytes and creatinine, ESR, fasting blood sugar, liver function tests, serum protein with immunoelectrophoresis, and urinalysis.

### D. Additional workup
guided by history and results from initial workup: heavy metal screen (24-hour urine and serum), urine porphyrins, urine amino acids, fecal fat, serum B12, serum folate, and CSF studies.

### E. EMG
is useful in distinguishing a neuropathy from a myopathy. This can be difficult to perform in the very young.

### F. NCV
determines the pattern of involvement (motor or sensory), type of involvement (axonal or demyelinating), and

degree of involvement and progression (on serial studies). Again, accurate studies may be difficult to perform in the very young.

G. **Muscle biopsy** in the setting of a peripheral neuropathy generally shows denervation.

H. **Nerve biopsy** (e.g., sural nerve) provides a specimen for selected studies. Often the findings are nonspecific, but in some cases nerve biopsies are diagnostic.

## II. HEREDITARY MOTOR AND SENSORY NEUROPATHIES

A. **HMSN type I** (Charcot-Marie-Tooth disease, peroneal muscular atrophy)

1. Segmental demyelinating and remyelinating neuropathy resulting in hypertrophic peripheral nerves. Autopsy studies show the anterior and posterior nerve roots, anterior horn cells, posterior columns, and spinocerebellar tracts have degenerative changes.

2. Autosomal dominant inheritance with variable clinical expression from nearly normal to wheelchair-dependent. HMSN-I comprises 51% of all genetically transmitted childhood peripheral neuropathies. The gene is located on chromosome 17.

3. Features
   a. **Orthopedic deformities.** Pes cavus, hammertoes, and elevation of the arch due to weakness of the dorsiflexors, everters, and intrinsic musculature of the foot. This is the most common reason for seeking medical attention. Skeletal deformities, scoliosis, kyphoscoliosis, and lordosis develop in up to 20% of patients.
   b. **DTR.** An absent or diminished ankle jerk. Areflexia may progress to involve the upper extremities.
   c. **Sensory loss.** Mild loss of vibration and position sense.
   d. Calf wasting (peroneal muscular atrophy).
   e. Enlarged, firm peripheral nerves are apparent in up to 25% of children.

4. **Course.** Onset is usually in the first or second decade. HMSN-I rarely presents in infancy (consider a diagnosis of HMSN-III). This is a slowly progressive disease that may arrest spontaneously.

5. Diagnosis
   a. Positive family history.
   b. **NCV.** Decreased motor and sensory nerve conduction velocities.
   c. **Nerve biopsy.** Segmental demyelination and remyelination with axonal atrophy, onion bulb formation, hypertrophy in myelinated fibers, and increased endoneural collagen.
   d. **Roussy-Lévy syndrome** is a subset of HMSN-I and is characterized by ataxic gait and a static tremor of the arms in addition to the features noted in part 3.

6. **Treatment** is supportive. Physical therapy, appropriate footwear, and orthoses should be prescribed as needed. Foot surgery may become necessary. Triple arthrodesis for foot drop has been used with good results.

B. **HMSN type II** (peroneal muscular atrophy, axonal type).

**Type A (Lambert type)** has an autosomal dominant inheritance and **type B (Ouvrier type)** is autosomal recessive. Both are characterized by axonal degeneration. HMSN-II generally presents after the fifth decade and for that reason is not discussed further. Clinical features are similar to HMSN-I.

C. **HMSN type III** (Dejerine-Sottas disease, hypertrophic interstitial neuropathy of infancy)
   1. Demyelinating and remyelinating neuropathy.
   2. Autosomal recessive transmission with a high number of sporadic cases.
   3. **Features**
      a. Hypotonia and delayed motor development in the first year of life. Facial weakness with a pouting appearance of the lips.
      b. **Orthopedic deformities.** Clubfoot, scoliosis.
      c. Sensory loss in all modalities resulting in a sensory ataxia.
      d. DTR absent.
      e. **Ocular.** Nystagmus, slowed pupillary light reflex, miosis.
   4. **Onset** is typically in the first year of life. Ambulation is delayed, and as many as half of patients progress to wheelchair dependency.
   5. **Diagnosis**
      a. Inheritance patterns help distinguish this entity from early-onset HMSN-I.
      b. **NCV.** Slowed conduction of motor nerves.
      c. **CSF** protein elevation proportional to clinical weakness.
      d. **Nerve biopsy.** Demyelination and onion bulb formation (more extensive than that seen with HMSN-I), interstitial hypertrophy, and hypomyelination.
   6. **Treatment.** Supportive with physical therapy and orthoses as needed.
D. **HMSN type IV** (Refsum disease)
   1. Chronic progressive polyneuropathy due to the accumulation of phytanic acid related to an inborn error of metabolism that blocks the oxidation of phytanic acid to pristanic acid.
   2. Autosomal recessive inheritance.
   3. **Features**
      a. **Neurological.** Symmetric, distal progressive **polyneuropathy** involving motor and sensory fibers, anosmia, neurogenic hearing loss, **cerebellar ataxia,** impaired joint position sense and pinprick, and dysesthesia.
      b. **Ocular. Retinitis pigmentosa** (night blindness progressing to tunnel vision), pupillary abnormalities, and lens opacities.
      c. **Other.** Cardiomyopathy, skeletal abnormalities, and ichthyosis.
   4. **Course.** Onset is usually in childhood between ages 4 and 7, but may be delayed until the third decade. The course is variable. On a phytol-free diet, patients can do well. The cardiomyopathy may be fatal.
   5. **Diagnosis**

**a.** Elevated serum phytanic acid of 10–50 mg/dl (normal < 0.2 mg/dl).

**b.** Increased CSF protein (100–700 mg/dl).

**c. EMG/NCV.** Denervation, decreased motor and sensory NCV.

**d. Electroretinography** reveals both rod and cone abnormalities.

**e.** Fibroblasts cultured from the patient demonstrate reduced oxidation of phytanic acid. In utero diagnosis can be made by determination of phytanic acid oxidation in amniotic cells.

**6. Treatment.** Phytol-free diet (no animal fat, green vegetables, nuts, dairy products, coffee) and plasmapheresis.

## III. HEREDITARY SENSORY AND AUTONOMIC NEUROPATHIES.

This family of disorders is characterized by a loss of sensation resulting in an insensitivity to pain. As a group, these disorders are quite rare and only HSAN-I, -II, -III, and -IV will be discussed. The primary differential diagnosis in HSAN is Lesch-Nyhan syndrome, which is associated with self-mutilation from other causes. Treatment involves prevention of injury through the use of protective gloves and footwear. Educating the family, and the patient when the child is old enough, can minimize injury. Infections, fractures, and ulcers that develop in association with these disorders need prompt medical attention to avoid the need for amputation.

**A. HSAN type I** (hereditary sensory radicular neuropathy)

1. Autosomal dominant inheritance.

2. Symptoms may begin in the first year of life with subtle features, but HSAN-I is not fully manifested until adulthood.

3. Loss of pain and temperature sensation primarily in the lower extremities leading to foot ulceration and infection. Other sensory modalities may be affected.

4. Sweating is typically decreased.

5. Mild weakness and hyporeflexia in the lower extremities may be present.

6. NCV of sensory nerves is variably delayed.

**B. HSAN type II** (congenital sensory neuropathy)

1. Autosomal recessive inheritance.

2. Onset is in infancy or early childhood.

3. All sensory modalities over most of the body are impaired. Loss of sensation is most pronounced in the extremities.

4. Infants are hypotonic and DTRs are typically diminished or absent.

5. Muscle strength develops normally.

6. The corneal reflex is diminished and fungiform papillae of the tongue are absent.

7. Autonomic function is normal except for mild anhidrosis in the distal limbs.

8. Because of the marked sensory loss, self-multilatory behavior in early infancy is common. Excessive sucking and biting of the digits leads to ulceration and infection. Trophic changes in the skin are common. Fractures often go unrecognized. Affected children may engage in harmful and

painful activities to amuse their peers (touching hot frying pans, etc.). Intelligence is typically normal.

9. NCV of sensory nerves is markedly impaired.

C. **HSAN type III** (familial dysautonomia, Riley-Day syndrome)

1. Autosomal recessive disorder occurring almost exclusively among Ashkenazi Jews with an incidence of 1:10,000–20,000 live births. Some sporadic cases have been reported outside this population.

2. Initial signs are present at birth: severe feeding difficulty, hypotonia, irritability, lethargy, developmental retardation, and failure to thrive. Recurrent vomiting and frequent pulmonary infections are common. Many affected children die in childhood from sepsis, cor pulmonale, dehydration, or hyperpyrexia.

3. Profound sensory abnormalities are present with decreased pain and temperature sensation and diminished proprioception and vibration.

4. Severe autonomic dysfunction is present including temperature deregulation, postural hypotension, hypertension, excessive sweating, abnormal gastrointestinal motility, and decreased lacrimation (no overflow tears with crying).

5. DTRs are decreased or absent. Motor strength is normal although motor coordination is poor.

6. Emotional lability is common.

7. Seizures are present in up to 40% of affected children, often associated with temperature elevations.

8. Adjunctive studies include the histamine test and methacholine test. The histamine test is performed by the intradermal injection of histamine (0.03–0.05 ml of 1:1000 dilution). Normally this causes pain and the formation of a central wheal. In HSAN-III there is decreased pain and diminished wheal formation. The methacholine test involves the instillation of methacholine 2.5% into the conjunctival sac, which normally causes miosis and tear production. In HSAN-III there is no response. Both of these tests can be positive in other neuropathies so they are merely supportive and not diagnostic.

D. **HSAN type IV** (congenital sensory neuropathy with anhidrosis)

1. Autosomal recessive inheritance.

2. Onset is in infancy. The initial sign is often hyperthermia related to anhidrosis.

3. The hallmarks of this disorder are absent pain and temperature sensation, preserved light touch, anhidrosis, and mental retardation. DTRs are normal.

# IV. METABOLIC NEUROPATHIES

A. **Acute intermittent porphyria**

1. Autosomal dominant inheritance. The gene for the defective enzyme (porphobilinogen deaminase) is located on chromosome 11.

2. Ninety percent of patients remain asymptomatic. When symptoms develop they appear at highly irregular intervals. Barbiturates (through induction of hepatic heme syn-

thesis) and alterations in hormonal levels (pregnancy and menstrual cycles) have been identified as precipitants. Only rarely do symptoms develop before puberty; however, porphyria should always be considered in the diagnosis of acute neuropathy of childhood, in particular in older children. **Congenital erythropoietic porphyria** is noted more commonly in children, and causes a painful burning in the feet (not neuropathic in origin) and a hemolytic anemia with exposure to sunlight. It does not have any associated neurological abnormalities.

3. **Clinical features.** Autonomic dysfunction (hypertension, postural hypotension, tachycardia), gastrointestinal disturbance (abdominal pain, vomiting, constipation), mental disturbance, and peripheral neuropathy. Cranial nerve palsies of the facial and oculomotor nerves develop in some cases.

4. A predominantly motor peripheral neuropathy is often preceded by pain or stiffness in the involved musculature. The neuropathy is somewhat atypical in that it affects the proximal muscles more than distal muscles and the upper limbs more than the lower limbs.

5. **Diagnosis**
   a. CSF protein is normal or mildly elevated in contrast to the high levels of protein seen in GBS.
   b. Decreased porphobilinogen deaminase activity in RBCs and urine.

6. **Treatment**
   a. Avoidance of precipitants.
   b. Acute attacks can be treated with intravenous 10% dextrose solution or hematin.

7. Respiratory failure from weakened respiratory musculature is the most common cause of death.

B. **Abetalipoproteinemia** (Bassen-Kornzweig disease)

1. Defective synthesis of **beta-apoprotein**, which is necessary for the formation of chylomicrons, low-density lipoproteins, and very-low-density lipoproteins. The result is a deficiency of the fat-soluble vitamins transported by chylomicrons (E,A,K) and diminished plasma cholesterol and triglycerides.

2. Autosomal recessive inheritance. More common in Ashkenazi Jews and males.

3. **Onset** is in infancy or early childhood with predominantly gastrointestinal symptoms: abdominal distention, steatorrhea, diarrhea, and frequent malodorous, bulky, fatty stools. These symptoms abate somewhat with age, but most children remain less than the third percentile for height and weight.

4. **Neurological symptoms,** thought to be related to vitamin E deficiency, begin around the age of 2 with one third of patients demonstrating neurological sequelae by age 10. Neurological manifestations include mental retardation, delayed motor milestones, loss of posterior column function, decreased cutaneous sensation, hyporeflexia, gait ataxia, intention tremor, dysarthria, and progressive muscle weakness.

**5. Other features.** Orthopedic deformities (scoliosis, pes cavus), acanthocytosis, myocardial fibrosis, and pigmentary degeneration of the retina.

**6. Diagnosis**

a. Decreased serum cholesterol (20–50 mg/dl), decreased triglycerides ( < 30 mg/dl) and decreased vitamin E ( < 1.3 µg/ml). Severe anemia may be present in young children (hemoglobin < 8 g/dl).

b. Absent serum beta-lipoproteins.

c. Prothrombin time may be increased due to insufficient vitamin K.

d. Acanthocytes on peripheral smear.

e. Dense lipid droplets in biopsy specimens of bowel mucosa.

f. CSF is normal.

g. Abnormal SSEP, VER, and electroretinography.

**7. Treatment.** Low-fat diet combined with high-dose supplements of vitamin E (100 mg/kg/24h PO), vitamin A (200–400 IU/kg/24h PO), and vitamin $K_1$ (5 mg PO every 2 weeks) starting at the time of diagnosis. Early and consistent treatment has been associated with normal development into the third decade and reversal of symptoms in some cases. Untreated patients progress to death by the fourth or fifth decade.

**C. Familial high-density lipoprotein deficiency** (Tangier disease)

**1.** Disorder of lipid metabolism causing an absence of high-density lipoproteins and decreased low-density plasma lipoproteins, phospholipids, and cholesterol.

**2.** Autosomal recessive inheritance.

**3. Features**

a. Deposition of cholesterol esters in the tonsils, spleen, liver, cornea, and lymph nodes.

b. Retinitis pigmentosa.

c. Hepatosplenomegaly.

d. Peripheral neuropathy presenting as either a dissociated sensory loss with progressive, symmetric faciobrachial wasting and weakness, or as mononeuritis multiplex affecting all sensory modalities.

**4. Course.** Onset is variable. Symptoms may appear anytime from childhood to middle age. The course may be transient or progressive.

**5. Diagnosis**

a. Decreased levels of plasma high-density lipoproteins and two apoproteins of the high-density lipoproteins.

b. Low cholesterol level.

**V. TOXIC NEUROPATHIES.** Chronic exposure, ingestion, or drug therapy may cause the development of a toxic neuropathy. This should be considered in the differential diagnosis of neuropathy of childhood.

**A. Lead**

**1.** Usually occurs as a result of the chronic ingestion of a lead-containing substance, most commonly paint flakes. Other sources include: lead solder, lead arsenate, insecticides, eye shadow, incompletely glazed ceramics, and sniffing of leaded gasoline. Less than 10% of ingested lead is absorbed. Low calcium intake, decreased 25-hydroxyvitamin $D_1$ and constipation increase absorption.

2. The neuropathy is evident as lower extremity weakness.

3. Ninety percent of children with clinically evident lead intoxication develop an encephalopathy. Within the brain, lead affects the capillaries, causing extravasation of plasma that leads to neuronal degeneration, predominantly in the neocortex. Additionally, it interferes with the calcium pump, causing a decrease in acetylcholine release, and an increase in dopamine and norepinephrine release.

4. Other clinical features include: restlessness and irritability, nausea/vomiting, anorexia, and ataxia. With progression, papilledema, increased ICP, convulsions, and renal dysfunction may develop.

5. **Diagnosis**

   a. **Radiographic.** Lead lines in long bones.

   b. **Peripheral smear.** Microcytic hypochromic anemia with basophilic stippling of red blood cells.

   c. **Urine.** 24-hour collection with increased levels of lead and Δ-aminolevulinic acid.

   d. **Blood.** Increased serum lead level.

   e. Evidence of renal failure (increased creatinine, BUN).

   f. **EMG.** Denervation of distal muscles.

6. **Treatment.** Calcium-disodium EDTA or penicillamine, both of which work by chelation.

B. **Arsenic**

   1. Acute ingestion of a large dose (e.g., consumption of rat poison) or chronic poisoning, which is often intentional and homicidal (not often seen in children).

   2. Survivors of acute ingestion develop distal (fingers and toes) paresthesias and numbness which ascends, and associated distal weakness. Chronic ingestion is suggested by peripheral paresthesias and numbness.

   3. Other clinical features of **acute** ingestion include: abdominal cramping, diarrhea, nausea, diaphoresis, and tachycardia that develop within minutes to hours after ingestion. **Chronic** poisoning causes weakness, anorexia, vomiting, and progressive skin changes —hyperkeratosis of the feet, skin pigmentation, Mee's lines (white striae in the nails), and irritation of the mucous membranes.

   4. **Diagnosis**

      a. Blood and 24-hour urine levels of arsenic.

      b. Samples of hair (pubic if available) and nails.

   5. **Treatment.** Chelation therapy using British anti-Lewisite or penicillamine in the acute or chronic setting. The latter may not respond to therapy.

C. **Mercury**

   1. Mercury poisoning is uncommon in children. Exposure to elemental mercury as a salt or a vapor, or from contaminated foods (fish) or fungicides may result in poisoning.

   2. Distal paresthesias, progressive visual impairment, ataxia, tremor, impaired mentation, and dysarthria are the most

common symptoms.

3. Congenital mercury poisoning causes microcephaly, hypotonia, myoclonic jerks, and tremors.

4. Diagnosis is made by determination of increased urinary mercury, elevated CSF protein, and history of exposure.

5. Treatment with chelating agents is recommended, although this is not proven to be effective.

### D. Aluminum

1. The ingestion of aluminum hydroxide and aluminum resins (some infant formulas) in children who have chronic renal failure may result in the development of a syndrome similar to that seen with dialysis dementia, which has a known relationship with aluminum.

2. Microcephaly, developmental delay, hypotonia, seizures and involuntary movements.

3. Treatment in adults has included parathyroidectomy, chelation, and removal of aluminum intake.

### E. Thallium

1. Intoxication usually results from the ingestion of insecticides or rat poisons.

2. Acute symptoms are primarily gastrointestinal (vomiting, diarrhea, abdominal pain). High doses (8–12 mg/kg) may be fatal due to cardiac and renal toxicity. Survivors develop painful, burning paresthesias and alopecia 2–3 weeks after ingestion. Ataxia, tremor, and optic neuropathy often develop in affected children.

3. Diagnosis is by history and evidence of urinary excretion of thallium by atomic absorption or emission spectroscopy. Fatty necrosis of the liver may result in abnormal liver enzymes.

4. Treatment with Prussian blue (250 mg/kg) to bind thallium in the gut. Potassium salts displace thallium from tissue for more chronic cases.

### F. Glue sniffing

1. Chronic inhalation of glue results in the inhalation of *n*-hexane, hexacarbons, and methyl butyl ketone, which are converted to 2,5-hexanedione, a toxic metabolite.

2. A progressive peripheral neuropathy is symptomatic with sensory symptoms initially. With continued exposure, muscle weakness and wasting develop.

3. Diagnosis is made by nerve biopsy or a history of glue sniffing. Nerve biopsy shows giant axonal swellings with neurofilamentous inclusions, thin myelin sheaths, segmental demyelination, and variation in the diameter of myelinated fibers.

## VI. ATAXIC NEUROPATHIES

### A. Giant axonal neuropathy

1. A rare, mixed polyneuropathy characterized by ataxia.

2. Autosomal recessive inheritance.

3. **Features.** Ataxia, nystagmus, and kinky, tightly curled hair.

4. **Course.** Onset is in early childhood and the disorder is progressive.

5. **Diagnosis.** Nerve biopsy reveals decreased myelinated

and unmyelinated fibers with segmental axonal enlargement. The hair is the distinct and characteristic feature.
**B. Friedreich's ataxia** (see Chapter 15).

# VII. INFLAMMATORY NEUROPATHIES

**A. Guillain-Barré syndrome** (acute inflammatory demyelinating polyradiculoneuropathy)

1. Acute to subacute demyelinating polyradiculoneuropathy.
2. **Incidence.** With an incidence of approximately 1:100,000
   persons, GBS is the most common peripheral neuropathy of
   childhood. Onset is as early as 4 months of age.
3. **Pathophysiology.** Destruction of myelin with infiltration
   of lymphocytes and macrophages in peripheral nerves and
   nerve roots. GBS is thought to be due to an autoimmune
   process. Recently this has been confirmed by the identification (in some patients) of circulating antibodies that bind to
   myelin.
4. **Features**
   a. Progressive flaccid weakness involving more than one
      limb. It is usually more pronounced in the lower extremi-
      ties and is typically symmetric. Weakness may ascend to
      involve the respiratory musculature, causing respiratory
      compromise.
   b. Areflexia is most commonly seen, but reflexes can be
      preserved in some cases.
   c. Painful dysesthesias occur in some patients. Young chil-
      dren may not be sophisticated enough to express this.
   d. Autonomic disturbance (blood pressure instability, heart
      rate instability and irregularity, sweating, urine and
      bowel dysfunction) occur less often and to a lesser degree
      in children than in adults.
   e. **Miller-Fisher variant.** Ataxia, hyporeflexia, and weak-
      ness confined to the facial and extraocular muscles. This
      is seen in only 1% of pediatric patients.
5. **Course**
   a. Approximately 60% of patients report an antecedent
      viral (upper respiratory or gastrointestinal) syndrome in
      the month prior to onset of symptoms.
   b. Maximal weakness develops within 1–3 weeks. Half of
      patients become maximally weak at 1 week, another 30%
      by 2 weeks, and 10% by 3 weeks. Some of the remaining
      10% improve during the fourth week and some continue
      with weakness. If relapse or continued progression oc-
      curs after the fourth week, the illness is designated as
      **chronic progressive** or **chronic inflammatory** (or
      **relapsing) demyelinating polyradiculo-
      neuropathy.**
   c. Half of patients can be expected to develop some signs of
      respiratory compromise, with only 10% requiring
      intubation and ventilation. Where possible, measure-
      ments of negative inspiratory force and vital capacity
      should be monitored.
   d. Two thirds of patients make a complete recovery. In some
      cases this takes several months and requires intensive
      rehabilitation. In pediatric series, about 25% of patients

have been left with a persistent deficit.

**6. Diagnosis**
   **a.** History and neurological examination.
   **b. CSF.** Increased protein with no or few cells. Protein can be normal in the first week.
   **c. Neurophysiology.** Decreased amplitude of muscle action potential, conduction block, and irregular abnormalities in nerve conduction. These changes may not be apparent until after the first week and reflect the multifocal demyelinating polyneuropathy.
   **d.** Elevated titers for infection may be demonstrated in some patients (e.g., CMV).
   **e. Differential diagnosis.** Botulism (often a history of eating raw honey) and toxic or metabolic neuropathy are the most important differential diagnoses. Viral myositis can be differentiated by an elevated CPK. Poliomyelitis is usually accompanied by a febrile illness. Spinal cord or cerebellar pathology generally will have other associated presenting symptoms.

**7. Treatment**
   **a.** Therapy is primarily supportive. Ventilation as needed, nutritional support if required.
   **b.** Plasmapheresis removes circulating antimyelin antibodies and immune complexes. Treatment several times weekly has been shown to decrease the severity of the illness and shorten the overall course. In very young children this may not be technically feasible. Risks associated with this therapy include line sepsis and venous thrombosis.
   **c.** Prednisone in high doses (1–2 mg/kg/24h slowly tapered over 1–2 months) gives symptomatic improvement presumably by reducing the inflammatory process in the nerves.
   **d.** Azathioprine (2–3 mg/kg/24h decreased to 1.0–1.5 mg/kg/24h after the first 6 months) administered for 1–2 years in conjunction with high-dose steroids has been reported to be effective. The mechanism of action is immunosuppression.
   **e.** Intravenous gammaglobulin (0.3–0.4 g/kg/24h for 3–5 days) results in clinical improvement. The mechanism is thought to be through the competitive binding of administered IgG, thereby preventing binding of the antimyelin antibodies.

**VIII. NEUROPATHIES RELATED TO THERAPEUTIC AGENTS**
   **A. Isoniazid** can produce a distal mixed sensory and motor neuropathy through its interference with pyridoxine. The use of pyridoxine supplements decreases the incidence of this adverse effect.
   **B. Nitrofurantoin** can cause distal sensory loss, paresthesias, and slowed motor conduction velocities. There is an increased risk of nerve damage with the use of this drug in patients with renal failure.
   **C. Vincristine** can be associated with decreased DTR, sensory

loss, paresthesias, and weakness. The hands are usually affected first, followed by the feet.

**D. Cisplatin** can cause a sensory neuropathy and hearing impairment through a sensory neuropathy.

**E. Chloramphenicol** used in high doses for a prolonged period may cause optic neuropathy and a distal symmetric neuropathy.

# Childhood Headaches

Headache in young children is generally not a psychosomatic complaint. In adolescents and young adults, this may not be the case. A careful history and neurological examination are essential in all pediatric patients presenting with headache to rule out organic causes. In very young children who cannot yet verbalize, a history of head banging suggests headache and underlying causes should be considered. The causes and management of childhood headache are discussed in this chapter.

## I. ETIOLOGY

A. **Structural lesions.** Brain tumors, hydrocephalus, vascular malformations, CNS spread of leukemia or other systemic cancers. Focal neurological deficits, papilledema, macrocephaly, or cranial bruits may be noted. Pseudotumor cerebri should also be considered, although it is not technically a structural lesion.

B. **Infectious.** Meningitis, brain abscess.

C. **Refractive error.** Rarely is childhood headache due to an ophthalmologic problem, but it should be considered.

D. **Functional headaches** rarely occur until early adolescence. The history is usually quite distinctive from that seen with migraines.

E. **Migraine**

F. **Cluster headaches**

G. **Tension headaches**

## II. MIGRAINE (VASCULAR) HEADACHE

A. **Epidemiology**
   1. **Onset** may be as early as 2 years of age.
   2. Migraines occur in 2–7% of children, with a slight increase in frequency with age.
   3. After age 10, females are affected twice as often as males.
   4. A family history of migraine is present in over 90% of cases.

B. **Pathophysiology**
   1. Migraines are thought to be due to vascular changes in both the intracranial and extracranial arteries. The vasculature is abnormally labile, resulting in symptomatic vasoconstriction followed by painful vasodilation.
   2. There has been considerable speculation about the relationship of migraine to epilepsy. Eleven percent of patients with a primary diagnosis of epilepsy have migraine and 7% of patients with a primary diagnosis of migraine have epilepsy. EEG abnormalities in migraine are discussed below.

C. **Characteristics**
   1. Location is variable and the pain may be bilateral, unilateral, hemicranium, frontal or retro-orbital.
   2. Pounding, throbbing, pulsating, paroxysmal headaches which are separated by asymptomatic intervals.
   3. Associated features include nausea, vomiting, visual auras, dizziness, vertigo, photophobia, sensory or motor disturbance, speech impairment, agitated confusion, and im-

paired space-, time-, and body-image ("Alice-in-Wonderland syndrome").

## D. Diagnosis

1. Migraine in childhood is a diagnosis of exclusion. Care must be taken to rule out any intracranial pathology.

2. Careful history, general physical examination, neurological examination, and review of family history are essential. A positive family history of migraine is reassuring, but not necessary. Nor should a positive family history of migraine lead one to make a diagnosis of migraine without careful evaluation.

3. CT or MRI scan should be obtained if the presentation is not typical, if there is any concern for a structural lesion based on examination, or if there is not a prompt response to treatment. Radiographic evaluation should be obtained in patients with progressive or persistent deficits. It is not unreasonable to perform neuroimaging studies on all patients with severe headaches.

4. EEG is abnormally slow or shows some dysrhythmia in up to 60–80% of children with migraines.

5. CSF abnormalities with migraine have been described and consist of a mild pleocytosis, predominantly lymphocytes.

## E. Types of migraine

1. **Classic migraine.** Symptoms occur in two stages. The first stage corresponds to the initial vasoconstriction with visual auras, visual loss, blurred vision, and scotomas being the most common prodrome. The second stage begins with the onset of headache and is often accompanied by vomiting.

2. **Common migraine.** Refers to vascular headaches which occur with minimal or absent prodromal symptoms. Younger children who are not able to give an adequate description may inappropriately be placed in this category. A careful history will elicit information about visual changes or other symptoms even in very young children.

3. **Hemiplegic migraine.** Unilateral motor or sensory symptoms associated with a vascular headache. Motor involvement may be hemiparesis/hemiplegia, or a monoparesis/monoplegia (most commonly affecting the arm). Sensory changes are typically numbness or tingling. Associated aphasia or dysarthria may occur. If symptoms are transient, occur in conjunction with the aura, and resolve rapidly, they are referred to as Type I. Type II hemiplegic migraine is associated with prolonged deficits lasting into the headache phase and beyond. In the majority of cases, resolution of weakness and sensory changes are complete within hours to days. In rare cases persistent weakness occurs. A history of trauma is frequently elicited in patients with this form of migraine.

4. **Alternating hemiplegia.** A rare syndrome thought to be a type of complicated migraine. This typically presents in young children, often less than 3 years of age. Older children may complain of headache, with younger children behaving as though they have a headache (irritability and head-banging). Associated symptoms have included seizures,

dysphagia, and apnea.

**5. Ophthalmoplegic migraine.** An unusual entity which involves severe headache arising near the orbit with spread to the cranium. The headache is usually accompanied by vomiting. With resolution of the pain, a partial or complete third nerve palsy develops. The sixth or fourth nerves may become involved. The ophthalmoplegia usually resolves completely within several days. These cases have been seen more frequently in males, and the number of attacks decreases with age.

**6. Basilar artery migraine.** Migrainous headache associated with brainstem dysfunction. Most often seen in adolescent females. The duration of symptoms is generally less than 45 minutes, differentiating this from more serious entities presenting with brainstem signs and symptoms.

**7. Posttraumatic migraines.** See Chapter 19.

**F. Treatment**

1. Rest in a quiet, darkened room at onset. Routine activity should not be resumed until 24 hours after resolution of symptoms.

2. With onset of the headache, Fiorinal or ergotamine tartrate can be used. In some cases acetaminophen is effective.

3. Children with persistent migraines may require prophylaxis with cyproheptadine hydrochloride (0.2–0.4 mg/kg divided TID), propranolol (1 mg/kg/24h divided TID), phenobarbital (15–30 mg BID), or phenytoin (5–7 mg/kg divided BID). Calcium channel blockers have been found to be effective in some patients. Those that have been approved for pediatric use are cyproheptadine hydrochloride and nifedipine. Antidepressants such as amitriptyline or imipramine (10–25 mg QHS) may be useful in some cases.

4. An assessment of possible provoking factors should be made both at home and at school. Where possible, stresses should be eliminated or minimized.

5. Other precipitating factors include missed meals, hypoglycemia, lack of sleep, sexual abuse, and postexcitement letdown. In older children, illicit drug and alcohol use or oral contraceptive use should be considered.

6. Dietary adjustments, in particular the elimination of cheese (not including processed cheese), chocolate, caffeine, and nitrates can decrease the number of attacks in a significant number of cases.

**III. CLUSTER HEADACHES**

**A.** Vascular headache that is usually centered about the eye with associated vasomotor symptoms of ipsilateral lacrimation, conjunctival injection, nasal congestion, ptosis, and miosis.

**B.** Attacks often occur at night and last 15–90 minutes. The attacks "cluster" over several weeks and may not recur for months.

**C. Management** in the acute phase consists of sublingual ergotamine tartrate (1–2 mg) or prednisone (10–40 mg as a single dose). Prophylaxis with agents used in the treatment of migraine is useful for chronic cases.

  **D.** This entity is rare in children. Thorough evaluation should be performed to rule out any underlying structural abnormality.

## IV. TENSION HEADACHES

  **A.** These are described as diffuse, non-throbbing, dull, bandlike headaches, often centered in the nuchal or occipital region. While they may last for several hours, they are rarely disabling.

  **B.** Oftentimes they occur in association with stress, and may be entirely absent on weekends or during school holidays.

  **C.** The physician should determine whether or not there are any hazardous precipitating factors present (sexual, physical, or emotional abuse). After careful history and examination, treatment is primarily supportive. Parents should be instructed to assist the child in identifying and dealing with the underlying causes of stress. Acetaminophen can be used, although it may not be effective.

# Brain Tumors

Brain tumors are the second most common cancer of childhood after leukemia. The incidence of CNS tumors in children is 2.1:100,000 population. This chapter will cover the most common brain tumors of infancy and childhood, organized by location.

## I. THE DIAGNOSIS AND MANAGEMENT OF MASS LESIONS

### A. Presentation

1. **Infancy**
   a. Progressive macrocephaly across percentile lines, split sutures, and a bulging fontanelle.
   b. Irritability.
   c. Vomiting.
   d. Failure to thrive.
   e. Delayed or lost milestones.
   f. Papilledema
   g. Blindness.
   h. Focal neurological deficits.
   i. Seizures.

2. **Older children**
   a. Headache.
   b. Visual complaints (diploplia, blurring, decreased visual acuity).
   c. Vomiting.
   d. Frequent falling, clumsiness.
   e. Weight loss.
   f. Seizures.

### B. Diagnosis

1. Neurological examination.
2. Radiographic workup.
   a. CT (+/-C). Steroids given prior to administration of contrast may alter enhancement.
   b. MRI (+/-G).
   c. Angiography.

### C. **Hydrocephalus** is a problem that occurs with many childhood brain tumors. If shunt placement becomes necessary and the tumor involves the CSF pathways, there is always concern for tumor seeding.

### D. Surgical resection plays a prominent role in the management of childhood brain tumors and is discussed under individual tumor types.

### E. Postoperative radiographic workup to assess extent of tumor resection should be obtained within 72 hours after surgery to avoid surgical artifact that has been reported to last up to 6 months.

### F. Adjuvant therapy is indicated in a variety of brain tumors. The effects of radiation therapy on the developing CNS are clearly deleterious. Children under the age of 3 are especially vulnerable. Additionally, the risk of radiation-induced tumors cannot be overlooked. Chemotherapy can cause a variety of systemic effects (immunosuppression, renal toxicity,

ototoxicity, etc), depending on the agent used. Chemotherapy may also damage the developing nervous system, but currently there is no direct evidence to support this concern.

## II. INFRATENTORIAL BRAIN TUMORS.
About 60% of brain tumors in children are located infratentorially, as compared with adult brain tumors, which are primarily located in the supratentorial compartment.

### A. Medulloblastoma

1. Categorized as a primitive neuroectodermal tumor.
2. Most common brain tumor of childhood in most series. Seventy percent of these tumors present before the age of 8. They are slightly more common in males than in females.
3. Arises from the multipotential external granule cell.
4. **Presentation**
   a. Increased ICP. Headache, vomiting, irritability, papilledema, macrocephaly.
   b. Ataxia.
5. **Examination**
   a. Macrocephaly (prior to suture closure).
   b. Papilledema.
   c. Sixth nerve palsy.
   d. Head tilt.
   e. Ataxia.
   f. Dysmetria.
6. **Workup**
   a. **CT scan (+/-C).** Medulloblastomas are typically midline high-density lesions in the region of the fourth ventricle that enhance homogeneously. Obstructive hydrocephalus is frequently present. As they arise in the inferior medullary velum, they fill the fourth ventricle and may invade the vermis, cerebellar hemispheres, or brainstem.
   b. **MRI (+/-G).** Further delineates the anatomy of the tumor and the relationship of surrounding structures.
7. **Management**
   a. **Preoperative.** Diversion of CSF (temporary or permanent) prior to tumor resection is a controversial issue. The risks of shunting include extracranial tumor spread and upward herniation, as well as the usual risks of shunt placement (see Chapter 13). About 40% of patients go on to require permanent CSF diversion even after gross total tumor resection.
   b. The goal of surgery is gross total resection where possible.
   c. Postoperatively, a CT scan (+/-C) or MRI scan (+/-G) should be obtained to assess the extent of surgical resection.
8. **Pathology.** Medulloblastomas are highly cellular tumors comprised of poorly differentiated neuroepithelial cells with small round nuclei. Mitotic figures are common. The cytoplasm is scanty. Other common features are the presence of Homer-Wright rosettes and multinucleated tumor cells. GFAP and AFP stains are negative.
9. **Adjuvant therapy**
   a. Medulloblastoma commonly metastasizes throughout the

CSF pathways. Complete spinal CT/myelography or MRI must be performed postoperatively to guide adjuvant therapy. At the time of myelography, CSF should be sent for cytology.

**b.** Extraneural metastases are uncommon, but sites include bone marrow, cervical nodes, and the abdomen. Bone marrow aspirates are usually performed to assess for spread.

**c.** Radiation therapy (craniospinal) is indicated in children older than 2 years. Chemotherapy is reserved for high-risk patients based on age, metastatic disease, and extent of resection.

**10. Recurrence.** Seventy percent of tumor recurrences appear within 2 years of initial treatment. Later recurrences have been reported. Reoperation should be considered in these patients, followed by chemotherapy (systemic +/- intrathecal). In most cases, patients will have received maximum irradiation. Survival in the setting of a recurrence is poor, with a median survival time of 20 months.

**11. Prognosis.** The 5-year survival rate is currently in the range of 60%. Patients who present at less than 2 years of age have a more dismal prognosis. The consequences of adjuvant therapy in survivors is not insignificant. Intellectual compromise, endocrine dysfunction, and neurobehavioral disorders are common.

## B. Cerebellar astrocytoma

1. Cerebellar astrocytomas comprise 12–28% of all pediatric brain tumors. Astrocytic tumors in general comprise one third of all brain tumors in children. More than 90% of these are **not** histologically malignant. They occur in the brainstem, cerebellum, and optic nerves.

2. Cerebellar astrocytoma is second in frequency to medulloblastoma.

3. The mean age of presentation is 9 years.

4. **Presentation**

   **a.** Signs of increased ICP from obstructive hydrocephalus related to tumor mass.

   **b.** Slow growth may cause symptoms to be intermittent in nature, with recurrent headaches or vomiting.

   **c.** Headaches tend to be frontal initially, progressing to suboccipital. They may be described as neck pain related to tonsillar herniation.

   **d.** Ataxia.

   **e.** Clumsiness.

5. **Examination**

   **a.** Nystagmus.

   **b.** Sixth nerve palsy.

   **c.** Papilledema.

   **d.** Gait disturbance.

   **e.** Dysmetria.

6. **Workup**

   **a. CT scan (+/-C).** These tumors arise medially in the vermis or in the hemisphere. Three basic patterns occur: solid tumor, primarily solid tumor with small cysts, and cystic mass with a mural nodule. One third of the tumors are cystic. Calcification may be present. Cerebellar astrocytomas tend to be hypodense midline masses that enhance uniformly or hypodense masses within the cerebellar hemisphere. The latter tend to be of the cystic variety and a mural nodule may be identified. Usually the cyst wall does not enhance and is composed of gliotic tissue; if enhancement occurs, it is likely to be an active tumor.

    **b. MRI (+/-G)** is helpful in defining the anatomy and evaluating the involvement of the brainstem in particular.

  **7. Management**

    **a. Preoperative.** CSF diversion, if necessary, can be accomplished preoperatively or postoperatively with EVD or shunting. About one third of patients with cerebellar astrocytomas will go on to require permanent CSF diversion.

    **b.** Gross total resection can usually be accomplished unless the tumor is adherent to the brainstem.

    **c.** Postoperative imaging should be obtained to assess the extent of tumor resection.

  **8. Pathology.** The most common histological type is the pilocytic astrocytoma, characterized by a biphasic arrangement of cells with oval nuclei and elongated bipolar or unipolar processes. In addition there are more loosely structured areas composed of astrocytes with small round or oval nuclei and small perikaryon from which arise delicate stellate processes. Other features include Rosenthal fibers and intracytoplasmic eosinophilic collections. Leptomeningeal involvement is common. The presence of mitoses does not suggest anaplasia. In children, malignant astrocytomas of the cerebellum occur only rarely.

  **9. Adjuvant therapy.** At present, no adjuvant therapy is uniformly recommended for benign cerebellar astrocytoma. In partial resections, some advocate the treatment with radiation therapy.

  **10. Recurrence.** Radiation therapy at the time of recurrence is an option. Reoperation should be considered. Malignant transformation of tumors previously irradiated has been reported.

  **11. Prognosis.** Gross total resection of a benign cystic astrocytoma has an 80–90% chance of cure. Partial resection is associated with recurrence in 3–5 years. Neurodevelopmental outcome may be impaired even in patients not receiving adjuvant therapy.

**C. Brainstem tumors**

  **1.** These neoplasms most commonly present in childhood and comprise 5–15% of all pediatric brain tumors, and 10–25% of pediatric brain tumors in the posterior fossa. They occur equally in males and females.

  **2. Presentation.** Upper cranial nerve palsies (oculomotor weakness, facial weakness), spasticity with or without motor weakness, and less commonly, lower cranial nerve palsies (change in speech, difficulty swallowing). Progression is usually rapid and tumors may be quite large at the time of initial presentation. Brainstem tumors may obstruct CSF outflow and present with signs and symptoms of increased ICP.

3. **Workup**
   a. **CT scan (+/-C).** Findings may be subtle with fattening of the brainstem or pons, or more obvious with hypodensity of the brainstem or frank cysts. Some tumors have an exophytic component.
   b. **MRI scan (+/-G)** is particularly helpful in clarifying the relationship of the tumor to the brainstem. The extent of tumor spread may be clearly seen.
   c. Not all brainstem tumors enhance with contrast on CT or MRI.

4. **Tumor types.** Brainstem tumors have been divided into five different groups based on their location and pattern of growth. The most common form is **diffuse,** accounting for 70% of these lesions. **Focal, cystic, exophytic,** and **cervicomedullary** tumors are the remaining types. The type and location of the tumor are the most significant prognostic indicators.

5. **Pathology.** Most brainstem tumors are fibrillary astrocytomas. The majority (60%) develop anaplastic changes consistent with glioblastoma multiforme. They most commonly arise in the pons and spread in an infiltrative pattern.

6. **Management**
   a. Steroids play a significant palliative role in the management of brainstem tumors.
   b. Obstructive hydrocephalus may necessitate shunt placement.
   c. Radiographically diagnosed brainstem tumors may be treated with radiation and chemotherapy without tissue diagnosis.
   d. The role of open and stereotactic biopsy is controversial. Biopsy can be accomplished, but not without significant risk. Sampling error in these lesions may be particularly high because of variable histological appearance throughout the tumor. In any case, management is not significantly changed, regardless of the histological type. Knowledge of histology is useful primarily for prediction of outcome.
   e. Surgical excision has been proven beneficial only in cases of focal or cystic low-grade gliomas in the brainstem or cervicomedullary junction. Complete excision is not the goal of surgery, but rather a 50–80% reduction in tumor bulk for optimal adjuvant therapeutic effect. Intraoperative brainstem evoked potentials are useful. Those patients with diffuse tumors have highly malignant infiltrating tumors that progress in spite of surgical intervention and should not be treated with operation.

7. **Adjuvant therapy.** Both radiation and chemotherapy have been used. Radiation has been proven to prolong

survival time to between 5 and 47 months. Of note, earlier reported 5-year survival rates of 41% were not in pathologically proven lesions and may have been skewed by the inclusion of benign entities. Chemotherapy has been shown to be useful primarily at the time of tumor progression.

8. **Prognosis.** The vast majority of lesions has a rapidly progressive course with death occurring in 12–24 months following diagnosis. Some low-grade astrocytomas have a more prolonged course with the potential for long-term survival.

9. Other lesions do occur in the region of the brainstem, but are less common. The differential diagnosis includes arachnoid cyst, epidermoid, hematoma (secondary to an occult vascular malformation), arteriovenous malformation, tuberculoma, focal encephalitis, infarct, and subacute necrotizing encephalomyelopathy. Unusual posterior fossa tumors seen infrequently in children include dermoids, epidermoids, acoustic neuromas, hemangioblastomas, meningiomas, lipomas, arachnoid cysts, and chordomas.

III. **SUPRATENTORIAL BRAIN TUMORS.** Approximately 40% of pediatric brain tumors occur in the supratentorial compartment. The **parasellar** region is the most common site (40%), followed by the cerebral hemispheres (35%), thalamus and basal ganglia (10%), pineal region (10%), intraventricular area (3%), and meninges (2%).

A. **Craniopharyngioma**
   1. Most common **suprasellar** tumor in children.
   2. Comprises 6–9% of all pediatric brain tumors.
   3. There is a slight male predominance in some series.
   4. Craniopharyngioma is rarely seen prior to 5 years of age.
   5. The peak incidence is between 5 and 10 years of age with a second peak in the fifth decade.
   6. **Presentation**
      a. Visual complaints predominate. Decreased visual acuity, bitemporal or homonymous hemianopsia, seesaw nystagmus, and papilledema may be seen on exam.
      b. Headache.
      c. Endocrine disturbance may present with short stature, obesity, urinary frequency, or amenorrhea.
      d. Not infrequently, craniopharyngiomas are discovered incidentally on radiographs obtained for other reasons.
   7. **Workup**
      a. **Neuro-ophthalmological** evaluation to include visual acuity and formal visual fields.
      b. **Neuroendocrine** evaluation to assess the hypothalamic-pituitary axis, the pituitary-thyroid axis, and the pituitary-adrenal axis. These studies are elective preoperatively, as they are likely to change after surgery. Postoperative evaluation is essential. Levels of GH, FSH, LH, TSH, $T_4$, and $T_3$ should be determined. Morning and evening cortisol levels should be obtained, as there can be a disturbance of the normal diurnal variation in serum cortisol. Rarely, a water deprivation test may be necessary to evaluate for diabetes insipidus.

    **c. CT (+/-C).** A low-density cyst of variable size in the sellar region with extension to the suprasellar region. There is often calcification within the tumor or at the rim of the cyst. The solid portion of the tumor varies in size.

    **d. MRI (+/-G)** is particularly useful to delineate anatomical details helpful in determining the surgical approach. Sagittal and coronal images clarify the relationship of the tumor to the internal carotid arteries. The cyst, which is rich in cholesterol crystals, is bright on T1 and T2 images.

**8. Management**

    **a. Preoperative.** Because these patients are often hypoadrenal, stress doses of exogenous steroids should be administered prior to surgical intervention.

    **b. Surgical approach.** The best approach is determined by the size and direction of tumor growth. A pterional or subfrontal craniotomy is usually performed. Patients with tumor growing toward the third ventricle may have obstructive hydrocephalus that often resolves after tumor resection. Shunt placement can be performed prior to tumor resection in selected cases. Stereotactic cyst drainage and biopsy can be performed; this approach may play a significant role in recurrence.

    **c. Intraoperative.** The proximity of tumor to the optic nerve and chiasm, carotid arteries, A1 segment of the anterior cerebral artery, basilar artery, and hypothalamus must be appreciated. While total excision is the goal of surgery, usually it can only be accomplished at the initial surgery. A subtotal resection may be all that can safely be accomplished.

    **d. Postoperative.** Initial postoperative management includes adequate steroid coverage until assessment of postoperative cortisol levels can be performed. A complete postoperative endocrine workup is essential. Postoperative imaging should be performed to assess the extent of tumor resection. Obvious residual tumor may be an indication for immediate reoperation. With total resection, diabetes insipidus occurs. It may be transient or permanent. Neuro-ophthalmologic examination should be performed postoperatively and then at yearly intervals.

**9. Morbidity**

    **a.** Visual loss can occur. Patients with preoperatively impaired vision of less than 1 year's duration are the most likely to improve postoperatively.

    **b.** Diabetes insipidus develops in the majority of patients and may be transient or permanent. This is readily managed with desmopressin.

    **c.** Corticosteroid deficiency may require long-term replacement with cortisone acetate.

    **d.** Hypothyroidism occurs in 60% of patients with a complete resection.

    **e.** Sex hormone replacement may be necessary at puberty.

    **f.** While GH may be deficient, growth can occur normally

without replacement therapy in some children. GH should thus be monitored to see if replacement is necessary.

**g.** The most profound postoperative morbidity is that associated with hypothalamic damage. These patients often become morbidly obese due to hyperphagia. They exhibit hypersomnia and lack of temperature regulation as well.

10. **Pathology.** Craniopharyngiomas are believed to arise from the squamous cell rests (Erdheim's rests) of an incompletely involuted hypophyseal-pharyngeal duct. Grossly, these are tumors of varying size. They may be primarily cystic, or partially cystic and solid. The cyst is filled with a yellow-green fluid rich in cholesterol crystals. Foci of calcification are often evident within the solid portion of the tumor. Histologically, the cyst wall is composed of a columnar or stratified squamous epithelium with a collagenous basement membrane. The solid portion is made up of epithelial sheets with pearly keratin formations. Adamantinomatous tissue (like dental anlage) is often seen.

11. **Adjuvant therapy**
    **a.** Radiation therapy is recommended in patients with subtotal resection, in those who have undergone a stereotactic procedure, and for the treatment of recurrence.
    **b.** External beam radiation therapy has been shown to be effective.
    **c.** Stereotactic injection of radioisotopes into the cyst has also been shown to be effective.

12. **Recurrence.** In patients who have not previously been treated with radiation, reoperation followed by radiation or radiation alone is recommended. In patients treated previously with radiation, reoperation and stereotactic radioisotope placement are the only options. Reoperation is associated with a higher risk, especially of hypothalamic damage, than the original operation.

13. **Prognosis**
    **a.** With gross total removal alone, the recurrence rate varies from 0–50%.
    **b.** In children, the 10-year survival after either surgery or radiation therapy is around 50%.
    **c.** Simple biopsy and radiation therapy are associated with a high recurrence rate and short recurrence-free survival.
    **d.** Many patients have endocrine deficits that are readily managed with replacement hormones.
    **e.** There is a risk of radiation-induced tumors.

**B. Astrocytoma**
   1. The most common tumor of the cerebral hemisphere in children. Optic nerve gliomas and hypothalamic gliomas also occur commonly in children.
   2. In children, the majority of these tumors will be of the pilocytic (juvenile) form which is low-grade. Only 4–7% of astrocytomas are malignant (glioblastoma multiforme) in children. Malignant transformation in benign lesions occurs rarely.
   3. Presentation varies with location. Optic nerve tumors typi-

cally present with visual complaints or exophthalmos. Lesions in the chiasm may present with diencephalic syndrome (profound emaciation with decreased subcutaneous fat, locomotor hyperactivity, and euphoria). Seizures, headache, vomiting, oculomotor dysfunction, and lethargy are common symptoms for these tumors.

4. **Workup**

   a. **CT (+/-C).** Low-grade lesions tend to be hypodense with rare enhancement. Anaplastic tumors may be hypodense or isodense with enhancement occurring in 80%. Cysts, mural nodules, and calcification may be seen (see sec. II. B).

   b. **MRI (+/-G).** Usually isointense to hypointense on T1-weighted images and hyperintense on T2-weighted images. More extensive edema may be noted on MRI than on CT scan. The majority will partially enhance with gadolinium.

5. **Management**

   a. Stereotactic biopsy is well-suited to deep lesions or lesions in functional sites.

   b. Surgical resection for lesions that are accessible should be considered. Lobectomy, where possible, may be curative.

6. **Pathology.** See sec. II. B.

7. **Adjuvant therapy.** Low-grade gliomas do not require adjuvant therapy even with subtotal resection. In cases of recurrence or symptomatic progression, radiation therapy may be used. Malignant tumors require treatment with chemotherapy and radiation therapy.

8. **Recurrences** may be reoperated or treated with adjuvant therapy.

9. **Prognosis.** Children with low-grade gliomas generally, fare much better than adults, with a 5-year survival rate of 83%. The actual survival rate varies somewhat with the tumor site, extent of resection, and age of the patient. Even low-grade gliomas can disseminate throughout the CSF and meninges over years.

C. **Primitive neuroectodermal tumors**

   1. Comprise about 5% of pediatric supratentorial neoplasms. The mean age of presentation is 6 years, with a slight male predominance.

   2. Most cases arise in the frontal or parietal region.

   3. Presentation is often related to increased ICP, oculomotor weakness, focal neurological deficits, seizures, personality changes, and ataxia.

   4. **Workup**

      a. **CT (+/-C).** These lesions are hyperdense with hemorrhage noted in 10% of cases, and cysts and calcification in 50%. Contrast enhancement may be homogeneous, solid, patchy,or along the rim.

      b. **MRI (+/-G)** demonstrates a well-demarcated mass with little or no edema. Signal intensity is heterogeneous and enhancement patterns are variable.

   5. **Management** is surgical excision with attempted gross

total resection.

**6. Pathology.** Small, round, blue cell tumors that are highly malignant. Areas of necrosis and hemorrhage are common. Variable expression of neuronal, glial, and ependymal cells occurs. Differentiation is associated with a better prognosis in contrast to those in the posterior fossa (medulloblastoma).

**7. Recurrences** can be managed with reoperation or chemotherapy. The prognosis with recurrence is poor.

**8. Adjuvant therapy.** Both radiation therapy and chemotherapy are utilized with some improvement in survival. Postoperative hyperfractionated radiation therapy and chemotherapy have resulted in some patients surviving 5 years after diagnosis. Morbidity in these cases has been significant.

**9. Prognosis** is poor, but survival is improving with new protocols.

## D. Ganglioglioma

1. A rare tumor composed of ganglion cells and glial elements.
2. Found more commonly in children than adults. In some series, they represent as many as 8% of the pediatric tumors. The incidence may appear to be on the rise simply because of improved diagnostic studies.
3. **Presentation.** Seizures, headaches, or behavioral problems. These are often noted as incidental lesions on studies ordered for other reasons.
4. **Workup**
   a. **CT (+/-C).** A hypodense or mixed density, well-circumscribed lesion that enhances variably. An associated cyst is present in 50% of cases. Calcification is seen in roughly one third of cases. Common locations include the frontal, temporal, or occipital lobes, the region of the third ventricle, and the cerebellum. If near the skull, they may erode the inner table.
   b. **MRI (+/-G)** shows a well-demarcated lesion that is usually hypointense on T1 and hyperintense on T2.
5. **Treatment** depends on location. Surgically accessible lesions should be resected. Total resection is usually curative.
6. **Recurrences** occasionally occur and may necessitate reoperation. Malignant transformation has been described.
7. **Adjunctive therapy** is not necessary unless there is histological evidence of malignancy. With malignant lesions and subtotal resection there is a high risk of recurrence. In these cases radiation should be considered.
8. **Prognosis.** Total resection is curative.

## E. Metastases
from neuroblastoma, nephroblastoma, and embryonal rhabdomyosarcoma are most common. Pulmonary metastases typically precede CNS metastases. Survival with metastatic disease involving the CNS is in the range of 2–20 months.

## F. Other tumors
occur, but are seen less frequently. These include meningioma (epidermoid, dermoid), lipoma, hemangioblastoma, hamartoma, oligodendroglioma, pituitary adenoma, pituitary carcinoma, and primary melanocytic tumors (malignant melanoma, melanomatosis).

## IV. PINEAL REGION TUMORS

**A.** Pineal region tumors account for 3–8% of all pediatric brain tumors. Seventeen distinct histological types of pineal tumors have been identified. Their presentations are similar. The clinical course is determined by histological type.

**B. Presentation**
1. Symptoms referable to increased ICP from an obstructive hydrocephalus: headache, nausea, vomiting, lethargy, irritability, and progressive macrocephaly in infants.
2. Third or sixth nerve palsy.
3. Papilledema.
4. Head tilt.
5. Ataxia.
6. Parinaud's syndrome (paresis of conjugate upgaze without failure of convergence).
7. Falling.

**C. Workup**
1. **CT (+/-C)** demonstrates the tumor and any component of hydrocephalus. Germ cell tumors tend to be irregular in shape and density, but enhance homogeneously. Teratomas have calcium, fat, and variable density.
2. **MRI (+/-G)** is particularly useful in defining the anatomy of the large draining veins with respect to the tumor for planning an operative approach.
3. **Markers** in CSF and serum can be diagnostic. In most cases LP is associated with the risk of herniation and should be done with great caution if appropriate.
   a. **ß-HCG.** A marker produced by syncytiotrophoblastic cells. It is elevated in choriocarcinomas, germinomas, and embryonal carcinomas with syncytiotrophoblastic differentiation. Simultaneous elevation of ß-HCG in plasma and CSF suggests a germ cell tumor.
   b. **AFP** is elevated in embryonal carcinomas and endodermal sinus tumors. Cases of germinomas secreting AFP have been reported.
4. CSF cytology can be diagnostic, particularly with pineoblastomas.

**D. Management**
1. The majority of patients has some component of hydrocephalus at the time of presentation. A decision regarding diversion of CSF must be made. If imaging studies suggest a germinoma, it may be preferable to perform ventriculostomy or shunt placement initially to study CSF markers. If another tumor type is suspected, CSF diversion can be performed in conjunction with surgery (ventriculostomy placement) or after tumor resection should hydrocephalus persist. About 60% of patients can be expected to need permanent CSF diversion.
2. Test-dose radiation for tumors that are consistent with germinoma can be considered. The disadvantage of this is that tumors other than germinoma can be radiosensitive.
3. The wide variety of histological tumor types in this region mandates tissue diagnosis for adequate treatment planning. Either stereotactic biopsy or craniotomy for tumor

excision should be considered.

4. Markers, if present, can be followed postoperatively and during adjunctive therapy for evidence of tumor recurrence.

## E. Pathology

### 1. Tumors of germ cell origin

a. **Germinoma** (pinealoma, atypical teratoma) is the most common pineal region tumor. The tumor has a male predominance and is geographically more common in Japan. It is highly radiosensitive.

b. **Yolk sac carcinomas** (embryonal carcinoma, endodermal sinus tumor) are tumors that demonstrate histological features of various stages of embryonic development, including the visceral yolk sac and amnion. These are aggressive, invasive tumors.

c. **Choriocarcinoma.** A malignant, invasive tumor.

d. **Teratoma.** Tumors composed of tissues derived from all three germinal layers. These tumors comprise about 2% of intracranial tumors in children and occur almost exclusively in males. They occur in a variety of forms.

   (1) **Mature teratoma** is composed of fully differentiated ectodermal, mesodermal, and endodermal elements.

   (2) **Immature teratoma** is composed of primitive elements, with embryonic histologic features from all three germ layers.

   (3) **Teratocarcinoma** is similar to the immature form, but it contains poorly differentiated epithelial areas as well.

   (4) **Mixed teratoma** contains elements of germinoma, embryonal carcinoma, choriocarcinoma, and teratoma within one tumor.

### 2. Neoplasms of pineal parenchyma

a. **Pineocytoma.** A benign tumor of the pineal gland composed of mature elements of the pineal parenchyma. It is a noninvasive, slow-growing tumor found equally in both sexes.

b. **Pineoblastoma.** A highly malignant tumor that is often placed in the category of primitive neuroectodermal tumors. This is the most common tumor type in children below 4 years of age. It may be associated with bilateral retinoblastoma, in a condition called **trilateral retinoblastoma.**

### 3. Other tumor types occur in this region, but are less common. These include pineal cyst, glioma, meningioma, hemangiopericytoma, hemangioma, chemodectoma, epidermoid, dermoid, metastatic carcinoma, craniopharyngioma, and melanoma.

## F. Adjunctive therapy is required in most pineal region tumors except completely resected benign lesions. Radiation therapy is used in most tumors. Many of the malignant tumors with a tendency to spread (in particular, pineoblastomas and embryonal cell tumors) require spinal irradiation as well. Chemotherapy has been proven effective in some embryonal carcinomas, pineocytomas, and pineoblastomas.

G. **Recurrence** can be managed with reoperation and adjuvant therapy. Usually, maximal irradiation will have been given, which leaves only chemotherapy as a viable alternative.

H. **Prognosis.** Benign tumors with total resection and no need for adjunctive therapy have the best prognosis, with virtually 100% survival (dermoids, epidermoids). Germinomas have at least an 80% 5-year survival rate; in pathology-proven lesions it approaches 100%. Pineoblastomas have a very dismal prognosis, as do yolk sac tumors and choriocarcinomas, with a mortality rate near 100% at 5 years. The morbidity from adjunctive therapy is not insignificant.

# V. INTRAVENTRICULAR TUMORS

## A. Ependymomas

1. Neoplasms arising from the ependymal lining. They most commonly occur in the fourth ventricle.

2. Represent 2–10% of intracranial tumors in children. There is a slight male predominance. Twenty-five to forty percent are supratentorial, and 60–75% are infratentorial.

3. **Presentation.** Signs and symptoms of increased ICP due to obstructive hydrocephalus. Seizures are present in about one third of cases. Ataxia is seen primarily with infratentorial lesions.

4. **Workup**

   a. **CT (+/-C).** Usually isodense and partially cystic. Calcification is seen in 50% of these tumors. Enhancement is variable. Intraventricular, periventricular, and parenchymal ependymomas occur.

   b. **MRI (+/-G).** Nonspecific, heterogeneous signal on T1 and T2.

5. **Management.** Surgical excision with gross total resection is associated with an improved outcome. Recurrence can be treated with repeat resection or adjuvant therapy.

6. **Pathology.** A variety of pathological types is seen: papillary, myxopapillary (exclusively in the conus medullaris or filum terminale), and anaplastic. The vast majority is benign, but those in the posterior fossa tend to be malignant.

7. **Adjuvant therapy.** Radiation therapy improves outcome. Spinal metastases occur in 15–50% of patients and spinal irradiation may be necessary. Chemotherapy, in particular cisplatin, has been reported to be effective by some groups.

8. **Prognosis** is in large part dependent on location and degree of surgical resection. In some series supratentorial tumors have a significantly better prognosis than infratentorial tumors. Degree of resection is an important factor, with gross total resection associated with a 60% 5-year survival, and subtotal resection or biopsy a 20% 5-year survival.

## B. Choroid plexus papilloma

1. Benign tumor seen primarily in childhood. Twenty to forty percent are found in children under 1 year of age. Seventy percent are located in the atria of the lateral ventricles (left more commonly than right). They may also occur in the third and fourth ventricles.

**2. Presentation.** May be associated with functional hydrocephalus or obstructive hydrocephalus and present with signs and symptoms of increased ICP or seizures.

**3. Workup**
  a. **CT (+/-C).** Well-demarcated, isodense masses located intraventricularly. Calcifications are present in 25–80%. Enhancement is uniform. Extension outside the ventricular system suggests malignancy.
  b. **MRI (+/-G).** Intermediate signal on T1 and T2. Evidence of prior hemorrhage may be seen.

**4. Management** is surgical resection. Placement of a shunt may become necessary if hydrocephalus persists postoperatively. The mechanism for this is discussed in Chapter 10.

**5. Pathology.** Histologically, these tumors resemble choroid plexus. Choroid plexus carcinoma is rare.

**6. Adjunctive therapy** is necessary only in cases of carcinoma, which are very aggressive tumors in spite of radiation or chemotherapy.

**7. Prognosis.** Complete cure is the rule with choroid plexus papilloma. Choroid plexus carcinoma has a mean survival of 9 months.

# Skull Tumors

A variety of skull tumors present in the pediatric population. The vast majority are benign lesions readily amenable to surgical excision, which is both therapeutic and diagnostic. Dysplastic lesions, congenital malformations, and malignant lesions occur. The presentation, various types, and management of these lesions are reviewed in this chapter.

## I. PRESENTATION
    **A.** Palpation of an abnormal lump by a parent or pediatrician.
    **B.** Incidental finding on skull films.
## II. DIAGNOSTIC STUDIES
    **A. Skull films**
        **1.** Benign lesions are usually solitary, widen the diploic space, have sclerotic margins, and may be surrounded by prominent vascular channels.
        **2.** Malignant tumors tend to have ragged margins and are often multiple (> 6).
    **B. CT** or **MRI** to rule out intracranial involvement. In particular, lesions in the midline should be studied to rule out dermal sinus or encephalocele, and to assess for possible involvement of the venous sinuses.
    **C. Angiography** or **MR angiography** is appropriate for vascular lesions.
## III. BENIGN TUMORS
    **A. Epidermoid and dermoid cysts**
        **1.** The most common benign skull tumors of childhood.
        **2.** They arise as a result of intraosseous epithelial elements retained during neurulation, or from iatrogenic deposition of dermal epithelium. Proliferation, desquamation, senescence, and occasionally secretion from these epithelial cells produce a cyst.
        **3.** Histologically, epidermoids contain only dermal epithelium and connective tissue. Dermoids contain dermal epithelium, connective tissue, and dermal appendages (hair follicles, and sweat and sebaceous glands).
        **4.** On radiographic examination these cysts appear as small, round lucencies with sclerotic margins.
        **5.** The natural history is progressive enlargement.
        **6.** Surgical excision is recommended.
    **B. Fibrous dysplasia**
        **1.** An abnormal accumulation of fibrous connective tissue within the bones.
        **2.** The skull has a characteristic widening of the diploic space and thinning of the outer table.
        **3.** Cranial nerves may be compromised as these tumors enlarge. Progression usually ceases at puberty with completion of skeletal growth.
        **4.** Thirty percent of patients have accompanying long-bone lesions.
        **5.** There is a risk of sarcomatous degeneration.

6. A combination of cutaneous skin lesions, sexual precocity, and skeletal fibrous dysplasia constitutes **Albright's syndrome.**

C. **Histiocytosis X** (eosinophlic granuloma)
   1. Intraosseous granulomatous reactions with histologically prominent eosinophils and a large number of histiocytes.
   2. When multiple lesions are present it suggests a systemic disease such as **Hand-Schüller-Christian disease** or **Letterer-Siwe disease.**
   3. Radiographically they tend to have lytic margins. They may be tender to palpation.
   4. Excision of solitary lesions is frequently curative.
   5. Secondary invasion of the pituitary-hypothalmic region from lesions at the base of the skull can occur, and in such cases endocrine dysfunction (i.e., diabetes insipidus) should be ruled out.

D. **Hemangioma**
   1. Benign lesions composed of capillary or cavernous vascular channels.
   2. The x-ray appearance is a sunburst pattern.
   3. Tenderness may be present.

E. **Sinus pericranii**
   1. A rare vascular lesion that communicates with the underlying venous sinuses through engorged diploic veins.
   2. These lesions are fluctuant on examination and tend to decrease or increase in size with any activity that decreases or increases venous pressure.
   3. Injection of contrast material into the mass with x-ray examination is diagnostic.

F. **Aneurysmal bone cyst.** A benign lesion composed of large vascular spaces separated by trabeculae of bone and connective tissue.

G. **Osteoma.** A primary skull tumor composed of mature cortical bone with dense hyperostotic outgrowths arising from the inner or outer table.

H. **Chondroma.** A rare, benign tumor composed of mature hyaline cartilage. These tumors arise in the paranasal sinuses or the synchondroses. They carry a risk of malignant degeneration.

## IV. MALIGNANT TUMORS

A. **Chordoma.** Originate from intraosseous remnants of the notochord. In the cranium they are most common in the spheno-occipital region. X-ray studies show destruction of the skull base. Treatment is excision with adjuvant radiation therapy.

B. **Sarcoma.** Rare tumors arising from connective tissue elements and their products (meninges, tela choroidea, stroma of choroid plexus). Primary tumors of the skull are rare. Metastases to the skull from fibrosarcoma or Ewing's sarcoma occur. Treatment is excision and adjuvant radiation or chemotherapy.

C. **Leukemia** uncommonly has associated intraosseous lesions that present as multiple lucent lesions. Treatment is usually with chemotherapy or radiation therapy. Surgical biopsy

may be indicated for diagnosis in some cases.
**D. Neuroblastoma** may have intraosseous involvement with multiple, lucent lesions and suture separation. Chemotherapy or radiation therapy, or both, is the usual treatment. Surgical biopsy may be indicated for diagnosis in some cases.

## V. OTHER
### A. Normal variations
1. **Pacchionian granulations.** Prominent lucencies around the venous sinuses.
2. **Parietal foramina.** Prominent defects of the parietal bone through which emissary veins travel. Very large foramina may be the result of faulty membranous bone mineralization.

### B. Acquired conditions
1. **Cephalohematoma.** A subperiosteal hemorrhage that frequently occurs during the birth process. These lesions respect the suture line. They tend to grow larger and softer as the blood products break down. Complete resolution generally takes 2–4 weeks. **Cephalohematoma deformans** may develop when the hematoma calcifies. This mimics fibrous dysplasia on x-ray examination, but usually the deformity restructures and resolves with time.
2. **Leptomeningeal cyst** (growing fracture). Linear skull fractures in children may be associated with a meningeal tear that leads to an expanding CSF cyst. With resorption of the bone along the fracture line, the bony defect may enlarge and herniation of the meninges and brain can occur. Treatment is surgical. X-rays show lytic lesions. The dural defect is larger than the bony defect.

### C. Congenital
1. **Aplasia cutis congenita.** Congenital absence of the skin overlying the calvarium. Frequently this is associated with an underlying bony defect and a fatal chromosomal abnormality.
2. **Encephalocele.** A small encephalocele may be mistaken for a skull tumor on physical examination. These appear along the midline. CT or MRI clarifies this lesion (see Chapter 8).

# Spinal Cord Tumors

Spinal cord tumors of various pathological types occur in the pediatric population. Their diagnosis and management are reviewed in this chapter.

**I. CLASSIFICATION.** Spinal cord tumors are classified by location.

    **A.** Intramedullary.

    **B.** Intradural extramedullary.

    **C.** Extradural.

**II. RADIOGRAPHIC WORKUP**

    **A. Plain x-rays.** AP, lateral, and oblique views.

        **1.** Extradural lesions are most commonly metastatic disease associated with lytic and blastic bone changes.

        **2.** Intradural lesions.

            **a.** Interpedicular widening.

            **b.** Pedicle erosion or flattening.

            **c.** Scalloping of the posterior vertebral bodies.

            **d.** Increased AP diameter.

            **e.** Enlargement of neural foramina develops with intradural nerve sheath tumors, with dural ectasia in neurofibromatosis, and secondary to vascular dilatation related to AVM or intraspinal tumors.

            **f.** Abnormal calcification.

            **g.** Spinal deformity.

    **B. CT/myelography**

        **1.** Extradural lesions cause displacement of the cord and dye column.

        **2.** Intradural extramedullary lesions displace the cord and cause filling defects of the dye column.

        **3.** Intramedullary lesions cause widening of the cord and displace contrast laterally. In many cases they are accompanied by a complete block.

    **C. MRI (+/-G)** is the study of choice for the evaluation of spinal cord tumors. Appearance is variable depending on tumor type.

**III. INTRAMEDULLARY TUMORS**

    **A.** Intramedullary spinal cord tumors comprise 6% of all CNS tumors in children. They represent 31% of all pediatric spinal column tumors. Approximately one third of childhood intraspinal tumors are intramedullary, and the remainder are extramedullary.

    **B.** Fifty percent occur rostrally (cervical or cervicothoracic region).

    **C. Presentation.** Signs and symptoms may be slowly progressive over months to years.

        **1. Pain.** Local or radicular.

        **2. Motor dysfunction.** Often there is a history of falling, delayed ambulation, or refusal to walk or bear weight.

        **3. Sensory disturbance.** Paresthesias, numbness, dysesthesias.

4. **Bowel and bladder dysfunction.** Acute or chronic dysfunction. The latter is uncommon except with congenital tumors.
5. Cervical region tumors may present with head tilt, torticollis, and nuchal rigidity.
6. Progressive scoliosis may occur with tumors at any level, especially if there is associated tethering of the cord. It is more common in thoracic lesions.
7. Progressive orthopedic deformities.
8. Hydrocephalus with signs and symptoms of increased ICP can occur.

D. **MRI (+/-G).** Enlargement of the cord (focal or holocord) with a poorly circumscribed mass (hypointense on T1 and hyperintense on T2). Ependymomas tend to have better demarcation. Associated cysts and hemorrhage are common. Enhancement is fairly homogeneous. Differentiation between ependymoma and astrocytoma by MRI is difficult. Ependymomas occur more frequently in the caudal cord.

E. **Management.** Surgical excision is appropriate. In holocord tumors, attention should be focused on the solid portion of the tumor. Intraoperative US and monitoring of sensory and MEP are helpful.

F. **Pathology.** In children, **astrocytomas** account for 60% of spinal cord tumors and **ependymomas** account for 30%. A variety of other tumors is found in the remaining 10% **(drop metastases, congenital tumors, hemangioblastomas).** Both focal tumors and holocord tumors (60%) are seen. The majority of patients with holocord tumors have astrocytomas.

G. **Adjuvant therapy.** Since these tumors are rarely malignant, radiation therapy should be reserved for histologically malignant tumors and in cases of tumor recurrence.

H. **Prognosis.** Outcome is based on tumor type and preoperative neurological status. Since the majority of these tumors are benign there is the potential for cure. Malignant tumors have a rapid course with growth and seeding of tumor. Unless the duration of preoperative deficits is short, recovery of function cannot be anticipated. In cases of partial deficit, recovery of function can occur.

## IV. EXTRAMEDULLARY TUMORS

A. **Incidence.** Forty-three percent of pediatric spinal column tumors are extradural and 25% are intradural, extramedullary.

B. **Presentation** varies somewhat with tumor type and location.
1. **Pain.** Radicular or local.
2. **Motor dysfunction.** Can be manifested as refusal to walk or bear weight, delayed walking, regression to crawling, or falling.
3. **Sensory disturbance.**
4. **Bowel and bladder dysfunction.** Failure to toilet-train or incontinence.
5. **Scoliosis** or other spinal deformity.

C. Vertebral column tumors
1. **Eosinophilic granuloma.** Benign, lytic lesion composed

of histiocytes and eosinophils that usually presents in childhood. It is most commonly found in the vertebral body of the cervical region. There may be multiple lesions (See Chapter 25). These lesions are sensitive to radiation and chemotherapy.

2. **Osteoblastomas.** Benign tumors usually located in the posterior elements (lamina or pedicles). Pathologically these are composed of osteoclasts and areas of mature bone and osteoid. Both lytic and sclerotic changes are present. Excision of symptomatic lesions is curative.

3. **Aneurysmal bone cysts.** Benign, expansile lesions composed primarily of vascular channels. They most commonly arise in the posterior elements of the cervical or thoracic region, but may expand into nearby vertebral bodies. On CT (+/-C) these lesions appear as an intraosseous soft tissue mass with enhancement. Acute expansion may be associated with sudden neurological decline requiring urgent operation. Low-dose irradiation can be considered for residual lesions.

4. **Hemangiomas.** Benign tumors found in 10–12% of autopsy series (more common in females). They occur throughout the spinal column. On CT the vertebrae have a polka-dot appearance. On MRI (T1 and T2) hemangiomas have a mottled appearance.

5. **Ewing's sarcoma.** Malignant tumor that is usually metastatic from the long bones, but may be primary. Most commonly located in the vertebral bodies, but may extend intraspinally with spread through the subarachnoid space. CT shows bony erosion and soft-tissue mass. With MRI these lesions have a low signal intensity on T1 and a high signal intensity on T2.

6. **Chordoma.** Malignant tumor that arises from intraosseous notochord rests. Most commonly seen in the saccrococcygeal region. It is a lytic, destructive tumor. Surgical excision followed by radiation therapy is the treatment of choice. Recurrence is common.

7. **Neuroblastoma.** Neuroblastomas are the most common intra-abdominal malignancy of childhood. They can be highly malignant tumors or tumors that have converted to a benign ganglioneuroma. Less than 1% arise from the extradural space. Others arise in the sympathetic chain and grow through the neural foramen. Prognosis is related to tumor type, age at onset, and stage of disease. Surgery for decompression of the spinal cord is appropriate.

8. **Others.** Ganglioneuroma, osteogenic sarcoma.

D. **Intradural extramedullary tumors** are uncommon in children.

1. **Nerve sheath tumors**
   a. Neurofibromas and schwannomas.
   b. Usually occur in the setting of neurofibromatosis.
   c. In the pediatric population these are more common in males.
   d. CT demonstrates an extramedullary soft-tissue mass.
   e. MRI appearance is highly variable.

  **f.** Treatment should be reserved for clearly symptomatic tumors that may be surgically excised.

  **2. Meningiomas.** Rare in children. Usually associated with neurofibromatosis.

  **3. Mesenchymal chondrosarcomas** are rare.

**V. CONGENITAL.** The majority of congenital tumors has an associated cutaneous change overlying the region, such as hypertrichosis, dermal sinus, capillary hemangioma, or lipoma.

**A. Teratomas**

  **1.** Can be located in the sacrococcygeal region or be intra-spinal (intramedullary or extramedullary). Sacrococcygeal teratomas occasionally present to the neurosurgeon with the diagnosis of myelomeningocele. However, these are usually managed by a general surgeon.

  **2. Pathology.** Composed of tissue from all three germinal layers. One third are anaplastic and may demonstrate local invasion and metastases.

  **3. Treatment** is surgical. Resection is curative in benign lesions.

**B. Dermoid and epidermoid cysts**

  **1.** Congenital tumors that are more common in children than in adults.

  **2. Pathology.** These lesions arise from dermal or epidermal rests.

  **3.** Most common in the lumbosacral region.

  **4. CT and MRI.** Epidermoids usually follow CSF density and for that reason are sometimes difficult to visualize. Dermoids have the same radiographic appearance as fat (hyperintense on T1 and hypointense on T2).

  **5. Treatment** is surgical excision.

**C. Lipomas**

  **1.** Intramedullary lipomas not associated with lipo-myelomeningocele (see Chapter 8) are uncommon.

  **2. MRI** demonstrates a hyperintense lesion on T1 and a hypointense lesion on T2.

  **3. Treatment** is surgical excision, usually with a $CO_2$ laser. The interface between tumor and neural tissue is generally not well-delineated and subtotal resection should be performed to avoid neural damage.

# Vascular Diseases

Vascular disease is much less common in the pediatric population than in the adult population. The diagnosis and management of vascular disease in the pediatric population are reviewed in this chapter.

## I. ANEURYSMS

**A.** Intracranial aneurysms in children are uncommon. They account for 1.3% of aneurysms in all age groups; 80% of childhood aneurysms present in the second decade. There is a male predominance.

**B.** They most commonly occur in the middle cerebral or vertebrobasilar system. Twenty percent occur at the carotid bifurcation. They tend to be larger in children than in adults.

**C. Presentation** is usually with SAH, headache, and the development of a focal neurological deficit.

**D. Diagnosis**

1. **CT (+/-C)** may demonstrate SAH, clot, or in some cases, evidence of a saccular aneurysm.

2. **MRI (+/-G)** is not useful in defining SAH, but signal voids may suggest flow through an aneurysm. MR angiography is helpful but routine angiography is still required.

3. **Angiography.** Defines the anatomy of the aneurysm, the relationship of the aneurysm to surrounding vessels, and identifies spasm.

**E. Management** is surgical in most cases. As technology improves, interventional neuroradiology may be appropriate therapy for selected cases.

**F. Outcome** is better than that seen with adults. Eighty-six percent can be expected to have good surgical results, with only a 3% operative mortality.

## II. ARTERIOVENOUS MALFORMATIONS

**A.** Congenital vascular malformations in which the arterial and venous circulations lack intervening capillaries, thus creating an abnormal connection between the arterial and venous circulations. These are believed to arise between the fourth and eighth embryonic weeks.

**B. Location.** AVM can arise throughout the CNS. Ninety percent of intracranial AVMs in children occur supratentorially. Most commonly they arise within the middle cerebral artery distribution. Spinal AVM presents rarely in childhood and will not be discussed further.

**C.** The incidence of AVM is estimated to be 0.14% of the United States population. While AVM is considered a congenital lesion, the vast majority of them do not present until the second to fourth decade.

**D.** Intracranial AVM and aneurysms are the most common cause of SAH in children (excluding normal birth and IVH in premature infants).

**E. Presentation.** Seizures, hemorrhage, headache, focal neurological deficits, and cardiac failure (in larger lesions).

**F. Diagnosis**

1. **CT (+/-C)** may demonstrate the tortuous vessels and any area of hemorrhage.
2. **MRI (+/-G) and MR angiography** define the vascular abnormality with areas of flow void and identify areas of hemorrhage. Areas of slow or no flow suggest thrombosis.
3. **Angiography** remains the definitive study for AVM.

G. **Management**
1. **Surgical.** Location and size are the predominant determinants of whether surgical excision should be attempted.
2. **Embolization** may be the sole treatment or may be performed in conjunction with surgery.
3. **Gamma knife.** Deep lesions of less than 2 cm in size may be appropriate for this therapy. It is reserved for the patient older than 4 years of age because of the potential risk of radiation damage to the developing CNS and the technical difficulties involved.
4. **Hydrocephalus** can develop following hemorrhage and may require shunt placement.
5. Anticonvulsants can be required, since the development of seizures is not uncommon, especially in cases that are not surgically excised.
6. Follow-up angiography after any therapy is required to ensure total excision.

H. **Prognosis**
1. Untreated AVM in children can be expected to rehemorrhage at a rate of 0.5 to 3.2% per year (up to 32% in 10 years).
2. Children have a higher risk of hemorrhage (77%) than do adults (68%).
3. Mortality from hemorrhage is in the range of 25%.
4. Sixty percent of children operated on for AVM can be expected to make a complete recovery. Thirty percent will have focal deficits, epilepsy, or mild retardation. The surgical mortality rate is slightly less than 10%, with the majority of these cases having significant preoperative deficits.

## III. VEIN OF GALEN MALFORMATION
A. Rare vascular malformation that is essentially a venous varix or aneurysm of the vein of Galen fed by numerous aberrant branches from the carotid or vertebrobasilar systems. Additional AVM can be present within the feeding vasculature of the primary lesion.

B. **Presentation**
1. **Neonates.** Congestive heart failure, cranial bruit, failure to thrive.
2. **Infants.** Hydrocephalus, seizures, cranial bruit, congestive heart failure.
3. **Children.** Headaches, hydrocephalus, SAH.

C. **Diagnosis**
1. **CT (+/-C)** will usually demonstrate an abnormality in the region of the vein of Galen. Hydrocephalus can be present.
2. **MRI (+/-G)** and **MR angiography** can be diagnostic.
3. **Angiography** defines the vascular anatomy and identifies the number and extent of feeding vessels.

D. **Management**
1. Interventional radiology for embolization of feeding ves-

sels. This should be accomplished in a number of settings over time.

  2. Direct surgical obliteration.
  3. A combination of interventional radiology and direct surgical obliteration.
  4. The development of hydrocephalus may necessitate shunt placement.

  **E. Outcome**
  1. There is significant morbidity and mortality associated with all forms of treatment. Mortality is probably in the range of 30–40% and higher (60–80%) in neonates with heart failure.
  2. Progressive deterioration of cerebral function occurs as a consequence of vascular steal and ischemia.

## IV. CRYPTIC AVM

  **A.** Small angiomatous malformations (arteriovenous malformations, venous angiomas, telangiectasias, cavernous hemangiomas) that are not visible on angiography. They can be seen on CT and MRI.
  **B.** Tend to occur in younger individuals.
  **C. Presentation.** These malformations may be seizure foci, sources of hemorrhage with headache and focal neurological deficit, or incidental findings at autopsy.
  **D. Management** is dependent on location, size, and symptoms. In noneloquent areas they are probably best removed to prevent rehemorrhage.

## V. MOYAMOYA DISEASE ([Japanese] "hazy," "puff of smoke")

  **A.** A rare vascular abnormality with progressive stenosis or occlusion of cerebral vessels as a consequence of fibrous thickening and hyperplasia of the intima. As a result, a fine network of collateral vessels develops at the base of the brain, hence the name **moyamoya**. The carotid circulation is more commonly involved than the vertebrobasilar vessels.
  **B.** Initially thought to be geographically limited to Japan, this entity is now recognized throughout the world. It occurs in females 1.5 times as often as in males.
  **C.** The etiology has been variously described as a congenital lesion, an acquired lesion, or a combination of the two. There is most likely a genetic component.
  **D. Associated conditions.** Arteriovenous malformations, intracerebral aneurysms, fibromuscular dysplasia, persistent trigeminal artery, Down syndrome, neurofibromatosis, syndactyly, sickle cell anemia, and cerebral radiation therapy.
  **E.** Four varieties of moyamoya diseaase occur: **hemorrhagic, epileptic, ischemic with infarction,** and **transient ischemic attack.**
  **F.** The juvenile form of the disease usually presents before age 10. Presentation in children is most commonly ischemic symptoms that are intermittent in nature: headache, hemiparesis or hemiplegia, monoplegia, sensory abnormalities, and speech disturbance. Seizures occur in some cases. Less commonly, children may present with intracranial hemorrhage.
  **G.** Workup with cerebral angiography demonstrates stenosis or

obstruction of the internal carotid artery, although the vertebrobasilar vessels may be involved, with an abnormal vascular network (collateral circulation) near the affected vessel. It is usually bilateral.

**H. Treatment**
   1. **Superficial temporal–middle cerebral artery anastomosis.** Technically very difficult in pediatric patients; usually reserved for older patients.
   2. **Encephalomyosynangiosis.** The temporalis muscle is laid over the cortex to encourage vascularization from the muscle.
   3. **Encephaloduroarteriosynangiosis (EDAS).** The superficial temporal artery, attached to galea, is laid over a dural opening for vascularization of the underlying parenchyma.
   4. **Others.** Cervical perivascular sympathectomy, superior cervical ganglionectomy, and omental transplantation.

**I. Prognosis**
   1. There is a mortality rate of 3% for juvenile moyamoya disease.
   2. Series of sympathectomy and ganglionectomy in Japan show a 61% improvement in children (compared with 47% in adults). These procedures have not been widely performed on children in the United States.
   3. Probably the most commonly used procedure for children in the United States is EDAS. With EDAS, an improvement in symptoms can be expected in a majority of cases. Early intervention before irreversible infarct occurs should be considered. Bilateral treatment is usually required.

# VI. STROKES
**A.** Strokes are far less common in children than they are in adults. They have an incidence estimated at 2.5:100,000.

**B. Etiology**
   1. Neonatal strokes are probably due to a wide variety of causes, including intrauterine events (arterial occlusion, infection), perinatal events (asphyxia, trauma, premature delivery), and systemic conditions (congenital heart disease, respiratory distress syndrome, disseminated intravascular coagulation, infection).
   2. **Vascular abnormalities.** Ruptured intracranial aneurysms or AVM, cerebral arteritis, atherosclerosis, moyamoya disease, or fibromuscular dysplasia.
   3. **Systemic abnormalities**
      a. Sickle cell anemia accounts for a large number of strokes. Twenty-five percent of sickle cell patients develop neurological sequelae, most by the age of 10.
      b. Homocystinuria patients are prone to thrombosis.
      c. Cardiovascular disease. Cardiac tumors, bacterial endocarditis, and left-to-right shunts may cause embolic strokes.
      d. Leukemia.
      e. Venous sinus thrombosis.
   4. Migraine may be associated with persistent neurological deficits.
   5. Trauma involving the extracranial carotid or vertebral

artery with subsequent occlusion, thrombosis, or emboli often results in stroke.

C. **Presentation** is typically with a neurological deficit. Hemorrhagic strokes may present with seizures or a dramatic decline in neurological function.

D. **Diagnosis.** Examination followed by CT (+/-C), MRI (+/-G), and angiography. The underlying cause of stroke in children should be searched for and treated if found.

E. **Treatment** is controversial and varies somewhat with the type of stroke. Hemorrhagic strokes rarely require surgical intervention.

## VII. DURAL SINUS THROMBOSIS

A. Thrombosis of the dural venous sinuses is seen infrequently in children. When it does occur, it usually presents in children less than 5 years of age.

B. **Etiology**
   1. In neonates, compression and distortion of the sinuses (with molding during birth) may result in dural sinus thrombosis (usually sagittal).
   2. Infection from sepsis or as an extension of osteomyelitis, otitis media, or mastoiditis can result in thrombosis.
   3. Systemic disease causing severe dehydration.

C. **Workup. CT (+/-C)** and **MRI (+/-G)** may demonstrate fresh clot within the sinus. MR angiography can demonstrate lack of flow through the sinus quite eloquently. Digital subtraction angiography is highly demonstrative.

D. **Treatment** is aimed at the underlying problem, control of increased ICP, and prevention of clot propagation. The use of heparin, urokinase, and streptokinase has been reported, but there is considerable risk of hemorrhage.

E. **Outcome.** The mortality rate is approximately 30%.

## VIII. VENOUS ANGIOMAS

A. Abnormal clusters of venous channels.

B. They are diagnosed with increasing frequency with the availability of MRI and MR angiography.

C. Most commonly found in the frontal or parietal lobes or deep in the cerebellum.

D. These lesions are usually found incidentally. There is a small risk of hemorrhage, and they may present with this. Some may be the foci in epilepsy.

E. Observation is appropriate unless they are intractable seizure foci, in which case resection can be performed.

# Epilepsy

A seizure is a sudden, transient disruption of normal cerebral function as evidenced by involuntary motor, autonomic, sensory, or psychic behavior. Individuals who suffer from seizure disorders by definition have epilepsy. Epilepsy is a common disorder affecting between 0.5 and 1.0% of the population, with slightly over 100,000 new cases per year. The incidence rate in newborns is 5%. In children under 5 the rate is 5 times that of the general population (excluding febrile seizures). The classification, diagnosis, and management of epilepsy are discussed in this chapter.

I. **CLASSIFICATION.** Seizures are classified by their symptomatology. The classification is important because it suggests etiology, mandates treatment, and relates prognostic information.
   A. **Partial (focal)**
      1. **Simple.** No impairment of consciousness with motor, sensory, or autonomic manifestations. Combinations of these manifestations are referred to as **compound.**
      2. **Complex.** Psychomotor or temporal lobe seizures with impaired consciousness. Automatisms or psychic phenomena.
      3. **Evolving.** Simple or complex seizures may evolve into generalized seizures.
   B. **Generalized**
      1. **Absence.** Typical (petit mal) or atypical, such as Lennox-Gastaut syndrome.
      2. **Tonic-clonic (grand mal).** May be intermittent convulsions or status epilepticus. **Tonic** and **clonic** seizures also occur independently.
      3. **Myoclonic.** Single or multiple jerks of a muscle or muscle group. This is often found in association with infantile spasms and other diseases (Lafora's disease, ganglioside storage diseases, subacute sclerosing panencephalitis).
      4. **Atonic.** Loss of muscle tone with unconsciousness.
II. **SEIZURE SYNDROMES.** Some types of seizures have characteristic EEG patterns or other distinguishing features that have led to the definition of a variety of seizure syndromes. These categorizations are especially useful for therapeutic and prognostic information.
   A. **Breath-holding spells** (reflex hypoxic crisis)
      1. Vigorous crying and breath-holding causing hypoxia and cyanosis with a transient loss of consciousness. While not a true seizure disorder, these spells are often accompanied by a brief generalized seizure.
      2. Breath-holding is fairly common, with nearly 5% of infants engaging in this behavior. Eighty percent of cases develop between the ages of 6 and 18 months. They usually disappear by age 6.
      3. **Treatment.** Anticonvulsant therapy is not indicated.
   B. **Febrile convulsions**
      1. Criteria for diagnosis of febrile convulsions include the

following:

**a.** Age < 6 years.

**b.** Fever of at least $100.5^0$ F ($38^0$ C).

**c.** No history of **nonfebrile** convulsions.

**d.** No acute systemic metabolic disorder.

**e.** No neurological disorder.

**2.** The incidence of febrile convulsions is in the range of 1.5–4.2%. Sixty percent of children have their first febrile convulsion before the age of 2. They most commonly occur in association with temperatures over $102.2^0$ F ($39^0$ C) in the setting of otitis media or tonsillitis.

**3.** There is a positive family history of febrile convulsions in 40% of cases.

**4.** Febrile convulsions are defined as **simple** when they are generalized and persist for no more than 30 minutes. The term **complex** refers to focal convulsions that last more than 30 minutes or occur more than once over a 24-hour period.

**5. Treatment**

   **a.** Lumbar puncture to rule out meningitis.

   **b.** EEG is indicated if neurological examination is focal, or if the febrile convulsion was complex.

   **c. Anticonvulsant therapy**

      **(1)** Should be considered in children with persistent neurological deficits following febrile convulsions.

      **(2)** Children who have suffered a complex spell, have a positive family history of febrile convulsions, or who have premorbid neurological or developmental impairments should be considered for prophylactic therapy as well.

      **(3)** Prophylaxis should be continued for a minimum of 1 year without convulsions.

**6. Outcome**

   **a.** Recurrent febrile convulsions develop in up to 40% of untreated cases.

   **b.** Epilepsy is more likely to develop in children with associated risk factors. Children with no risk factors or one risk factor have a 2% chance of developing epilepsy, while those with two risk factors have a 13% chance. Risk factors include the following:

      **(1)** Complex febrile convulsion.

      **(2)** Family history of febrile convulsions.

      **(3)** Premorbid neurological or developmental impairment.

## C. Status epilepticus

**1.** Seizures persisting for more than 30 minutes or recurrent seizures without regaining consciousness for at least 30 minutes constitutes status epilepticus.

**2. Treatment**

   **a.** ABC. Oxygenation, blood pressure, and heart rate and rhythm should be monitored continuously.

   **b.** Blood should be drawn for baseline glucose, chemistries, complete blood count, and anticonvulsant levels.

   **c.** Intravenous administration of 10% glucose.

   **d.** Intravenous diazepam (up to 0.2 mg/kg over 1–2 minutes). Be prepared to provide respiratory support if respirations become impaired.

**e.** Lorazepam (0.05 mg/kg up to 2 mg) may be used as the first-line agent instead of, or in addition to, diazepam.

**f.** Anticonvulsant therapy should be initiated with either phenytoin or phenobarbital. This decision is based on the choice of a drug for long-term therapy. The loading dose of phenytoin is 10–20 mg/kg IV (not faster than 0.5 mg/kg/min in neonates and 50 mg/min in children). The loading dose of phenobarbital is 5–10 mg/kg IV. Then 5 mg/kg IV can be repeated in 30 minutes.

**g.** If these measures do not stop seizure activity, intubation and general anesthesia may be required.

**h.** Appropriate continued therapy should be selected.

**D. Infantile spasms** (West's syndrome).

1. Seizure activity characterized by a jackknife motion with sudden flexion and adduction of the limbs and flexion of the neck and trunk. The seizures tend to occur in clusters.

2. **Onset.** Ninety percent of cases develop in the first 12 months of life. Onset before 3 months or after 4 years of age is uncommon.

3. **Features**

   **a.** Half of children have evidence of a prior cerebral abnormality such as perinatal brain damage, infection, malformation, degenerative disorder, or biochemical abnormality.

   **b.** In up to 30% of cases, infantile spasms represent the presenting symptom of tuberous sclerosis.

   **c.** Metabolic disorders such as phenylketonuria should be ruled out.

   **d.** A causal relationship between infantile spasms and immunizations (in particular, diphtheria, pertussis, and tetanus) has been suggested but not confirmed.

4. **EEG.** Hypsarrhythmia, high-voltage slow waves, and random spikes.

5. **Treatment**

   **a.** At the time of onset, corticotropin (5–8 U/kg/24h IM divided bid) should be initiated and continued for 21 days followed by a slow taper.

   **b.** Clonazepam or valproic acid should be started while the child is still receiving steroids.

6. **Course**

   **a.** The onset of spasms is usually followed by a decline and then regression in development.

   **b.** Mental retardation is apparent in most children with infantile spasms (70–96%).

   **c.** Infantile spasms often abate by about age 3; however, a significant number of children go on to develop severe myoclonic or akinetic epilepsy.

**E. Lennox-Gastaut syndrome**

1. Characterized by a triad of mental retardation, slow spike-wave complexes on EEG, and seizures. The seizures are of several varieties (akinetic, atypical absence, myoclonic) and are often highly resistant to treatment.

**2. Onset.** Half of cases present before the age of 2. The remainder typically present between the ages of 3 and 5.

**3. Features**

    **a.** A triad of mental retardation, seizures, and slow spike-wave on EEG.

    **b.** Perinatal and postnatal brain damage and neuro-cutaneous syndromes are noted in 60% of cases.

    **c.** A history of infantile spasms is present in 20% of children with Lennox-Gastaut syndrome.

**4. EEG** shows slow spike-wave (1.5–2.5 Hz) activity.

**5. Treatment**

    **a.** Management of the seizures is typically very difficult.

    **b.** Clonazepam is often considered the first-line agent.

    **c.** Valproic acid is also effective and can be used in conjunction with clonazepam.

    **d.** ACTH and corticosteroids have been used with some success.

**6. Outcome.** Ninety percent of affected children are mentally retarded by the age of 5. Seizures are often intractable.

**F. Epilepsia partialis continua** (Kojewnikow's syndrome)

    **1.** Continuous jerks or clonic movements of the face or upper extremities; considered to be a variant of a simple focal seizure.

    **2. Onset** is variable.

    **3. Features.** Focal clonic movements of the face or extremities that are not associated with an alteration in consciousness. Postictal weakness is common and some patients develop a progressive hemiplegia.

    **4. EEG** is variable and may show focal abnormalities or have an abnormal background with diffuse and focal paroxysmal features.

    **5. Treatment** does not alter the course. Surgical resection of the foci has been largely unsuccessful.

    **6. Outcome.** Most patients develop a progressive hemiplegia and mental deterioration.

**G. Gelastic epilepsy.** Forced, paroxysmal laughter associated with a loss of consciousness has been reported as a manifestation of seizure activity. In conjunction with precocious puberty, a hypothalamic tumor should be considered.

**H. Benign Rolandic epilepsy**

    **1.** A benign partial focal epilepsy.

    **2. Onset** is usually between the ages of 7 and 10.

    **3. Features.**

        **a.** Episodes are characterized by a sensory event, often of the tongue. Dysarthria, drooling, or tonic-clonic movements of the facial musculature (hemifacial seizures) are common.

        **b.** In half of patients, seizures occur only in sleep, just after falling asleep or prior to waking up.

    **4. EEG.** Midtemporal or central spike foci.

    **5. Treatment** with phenobarbital, phenytoin, or carbamazepine is effective.

    **6. Outcome** is excellent, with 50% of patients becoming seizure-free within 3 years of onset and 75% within 5 years.

Mental retardation and behavioral and learning disorders do not usually develop.

## I. Benign occipital epilepsy of childhood
1. Seizures manifested by visual phenomena.
2. **Onset** is between 2 and 9 years of age, most commonly before the age of 5.
3. **Features.** Seizure activity manifested by visual illusions, hallucinations, or visual loss. Motor seizure activity (complex partial, unilateral clonic, or tonic-clonic) often follows. Most episodes occur while falling asleep.
4. **EEG** during eye closure demonstrates unilateral or bilateral spike-waves over the occipital and posterior temporal regions.
5. **Treatment** with most anticonvulsants provides good seizure control.
6. **Outcome** is good. Most cases abate by adolescence. Only 5% of patients have seizures as adults.

## J. Rasmussen's syndrome (chronic focal encephalitis)
1. Intractable focal seizures associated with focal cerebritis.
2. **Onset** is usually before age 10.
3. **Features.** Focal seizures associated with cerebritis, confirmed by histological examination of brain biopsy specimens demonstrating astrogliosis and perivascular lymphocytic infiltration.
4. **EEG** demonstrates lateralized spike foci with underlying slow wave disturbance.
5. **Treatment** with anticonvulsants is generally ineffective. Hemispherectomy has had mixed results.
6. **Outcome** is poor, with most patients suffering from behavioral disorders and developmental delay and regression.

## K. Landau-Kleffner syndrome
1. Complex partial seizures or status epilepticus with associated speech arrest and aphasia.
2. **Onset** is between 2 and 11 years of age.
3. **Features.** Complex partial seizures or generalized seizures with decreased speech and difficulty comprehending. The speech disturbance is often interpreted as deafness, psychosis, or autism. Fifty percent of children develop personality disturbance and hyperactive behavior. Liver biopsy demonstrates mucopolysaccharide-like inclusions in hepatocytes and Kupffer's cells.
4. **EEG** reveals multifocal cortical spike discharges predominantly in the temporal and parietal lobes.
5. **Treatment** with anticonvulsants usually is effective.
6. **Outcome.** Seizures usually stop by age 10–15. Language can remain impaired.

## L. Pseudoseizures
1. Hysterical seizure activity can present in patients with or without true epilepsy.
2. Pseudoseizures are often readily distinguished from true seizure activity. In some cases they can simulate real seizure activity. They are often brought on by suggestion, or can be induced. Patients do not harm themselves or become incontinent during pseudoseizure activity.

   **3.** Psychotherapy may be necessary for the management of pseudoseizures.

## III. MEDICAL THERAPY

   **A. Initiation of anticonvulsant therapy.** Anticonvulsant therapy is initiated to control seizure activity. A single agent should be administered and if adequate levels do not result in seizure control, subsequent agents can be added. Seventy-five percent of children with epilepsy can be successfully managed with monotherapy.

   **B. Anticonvulsant agents.** Indications, dosing, and common side effects for some of the more commonly used agents are briefly discussed here. Prior to prescribing any of these agents, the physician should review more specific drug information. Additionally, possible drug interactions should be investigated prior to prescribing other medications for children on anticonvulsant therapy.

   **1. Phenytoin**

   **a. Indications.** Partial and tonic-clonic seizures. Useful in status epilepticus.

   **b. Dosage.** 5–10 mg/kg/24h divided bid. Therapeutic level is 10–20 µg/ml.

   **c. Side effects.** Gum hypertrophy, hirsutism, and hypersensitivity. Toxicity is usually manifested by ataxia, nystagmus, and diploplia.

   **2. Phenobarbital**

   **a. Indications.** Simple partial and tonic-clonic seizures.

   **b. Dosage.** 3–5 mg/kg/24h divided qid to bid. Therapeutic level is 10–40 µg/ml.

   **c. Side effects.** Hyperactivity and irritability or oversedation.

   **3. Carbamazepine**

   **a. Indications.** Partial and tonic-clonic seizures.

   **b. Dosage.** 15–25 mg/kg/24h divided tid to qid. Because carbamazepine induces its own metabolism, the dosage should be gradually increased to maintenance doses to avoid toxic side effects. Concurrent use of erythromycin may result in toxicity. Therapeutic level is 4–12 µg/ml.

   **c. Side effects.** Thrombocytopenia and leukopenia are the most common adverse effects. At a minimum, a complete blood count should be performed prior to the initiation of therapy, 6 weeks into therapy, and periodically thereafter. Ataxia, nystagmus, and sedation develop at toxic levels.

   **4. Valproic acid**

   **a. Indications.** Tonic-clonic, myotonic, absence, and mixed seizures. Also used in the treatment of infantile spasms.

   **b. Dosage.** 20–60 mg/kg/24h divided bid to tid. Therapeutic level is 50–120 µg/ml.

   **c. Side effects.** The major side effect is a dose-related hepatotoxicity that can progress to fatal hepatic necrosis. Hyperammonemia and gastric discomfort also occur. Baseline and periodic complete blood count and liver function studies should be obtained in patients treated with valproic acid.

**5. Clonazepam**
    **a. Indications.** Partial, absence, and myoclonic seizures. Also used in the treatment of infantile spasms.
    **b. Dosage.** 0.1–0.2 mg/kg/24h divided bid to tid. Therapeutic level is 15–18 ng/ml.
    **c. Side effects.** Lethargy, behavioral disturbance, and salivation.

**6. Ethosuximide**
    **a. Indications.** Absence seizures.
    **b. Dosage.** 10–40 mg/kg/24h divided bid to qid. Therapeutic level is 40–100 µg/ml.
    **c. Side effects.** Gastrointestinal symptoms and, rarely, bone marrow depression or a lupuslike syndrome.

**7. Primidone**
    **a. Indications.** Complex partial and tonic-clonic seizures.
    **b. Dosage.** 10–25 mg/kg/24h divided tid to qid. Therapeutic level is 4–12 µg/ml.
    **c. Side effects.** Gastrointestinal symptoms, lethargy, and ataxia.

**C. Withdrawal of therapy** is a complicated issue; however, a 2–4 year seizure-free interval should pass prior to attempts to withdraw therapy. There is an increased risk of recurrent seizures in patients in whom seizures were difficult to control, if epileptiform activity is present on EEG when drugs are discontinued, and in developmentally or neurologically impaired individuals.

**D. Ketogenic diet**
    **1.** A diet restricting the intake of protein and carbohydrates with the majority of calories derived from the intake of fats. Supplemental vitamins should be administered.
    **2.** Based on the observation that ketonuria has a worthwhile effect on epilepsy.
    **3.** Used in the treatment of intractable seizure disorders.
    **4.** Adverse effects of this regimen include gastrointestinal symptoms (diarrhea, cramps, nausea) and symptoms related to hypoglycemia. The diet is not well-tolerated because of its composition.

**IV. EVALUATION OF INTRACTABLE EPILEPSY.** Intractable seizures are defined as seizures that are refractory to maximal medical therapy with multiple anticonvulsants in adequate levels and combinations thereof.

**A.** History, neurological evaluation, medication history, categorization of epilepsy, and determination of intractability of seizure disorder.

**B. CT** or **MRI** to demonstrate structural lesions.

**C. PET** may be useful in detecting functional abnormalities in the form of hypometabolism.

**D. EEG video monitoring.** Recording of seizure activity on video with simultaneous EEG recording to rule out pseudoseizures and to further categorize and determine the focus of seizure activity.

**E. Depth electrodes.** Stereotactic placement of electrodes bilaterally in the amygdala, hippocampus, frontal cortex, and in some cases, the occipital cortex. Following electrode placement, continuous recording from the electrodes with or without video monitoring to evaluate seizure focus. With depth electrodes in place, a thiopental sodium activation test can be performed. This involves the administration of intravenous thiopental under the care of an anesthesiologist until hypoxia, hypotension, or loss of the corneal reflex occurs. Normally, this will induce beta activity in the EEG. The failure to induce beta activity suggests focal cerebral dysfunction. Afterdischarge thresholds can also be assessed with depth electrodes to establish relative thresholds in homologous regions. The side with the higher threshold is thought to contain the focal pathology.

**F. Foramen ovale electrodes.** Invasive monitoring similar to depth electrodes with placement of the electrodes through the foramen ovale for the evaluation of temporal lobe epilepsy. Continuous EEG monitoring is carried out following electrode placement.

**G. Wada test (carotid amobarbital test).** Assessment of laterality of memory function and speech prior to temporal lobe surgery.

**H. Neuropsychological testing** primarily for baseline assessment. Patients with or without neurobehavioral problems are candidates for surgical therapy.

**I. Somatosensory evoked potentials.** Median nerve SSEP allows evaluation of the symmetry of the thalamocortical peaks in lesions thought to be near the somatosensory pathways. The abnormal peak is associated with cortical abnormality.

## V. SURGERY

**A.** Surgery for epilepsy in children is unique because of the effects of intractable seizure activity and operation on the immature, developing brain. The developing brain has plasticity that may improve postoperative outcome.

**B.** Surgical treatment for intractable seizures in children should be performed as early as possible. Uncontrolled seizure disorders in childhood have a negative impact on the development, education, and socialization of children. Further, it has been demonstrated that prolonged anticonvulsant drug therapy affects cognition, behavior, memory, and motor development in a substantial number of children.

**C.** Criteria for surgery
  1. Intractable seizures with a unilateral focus (temporal lobectomy or focal resection).
  2. Intractable seizures characterized by atonic episodes or partial seizures with generalization (corpus callosotomy).

## VI. OPERATIONS

**A. Hemispherectomy**
  1. Previously has been associated with a high morbidity, but currently is regaining popularity. A functional hemispherectomy consists of resection of the temporal lobe and central region, with sparing of portions of the occipital and frontal lobes after resection of their connections to the remainder of the brain.
  2. **Indications.** A substantial hemiparesis with intractable

focal or generalized seizures with a focus in the hemisphere contralateral to the hemiplegia.

3. **Hemimegalencephaly,** diffuse enlargement of one hemisphere, may be associated with seizure activity responsive to hemispherectomy.

4. **Complications.** Subdural hematoma, hemosiderosis (small, chronic bleeding from a subdural membrane), late encephalopathy, and hydrocephalus are the major complications. Bleeding complications are significantly reduced with functional hemispherectomy.

5. **Outcome.** In appropriately selected candidates, greater than 85% have a substantial reduction in seizures or are seizure-free after hemispherectomy. Additionally, about one third of patients will have an improvement in their contralateral hemiparesis.

## B. Focal resection

1. Surgical resection of the localized seizure focus. This may or may not be a structural lesion.

2. In children, common structural lesions may be tumor, cavernous angioma, Sturge-Weber anomaly, porencephalic cyst, cortical dysplasia, or arachnoid cyst.

3. As children usually cannot be operated on while awake, preoperative assessment with monitored epidural electrodes and intraoperative SSEP can be used to avoid damage to functionally important areas.

4. **Complications.** The major complication is a persisting focal neurological deficit such as hemiparesis or aphasia.

5. **Outcome.** Fifty to sixty-five percent of appropriately selected patients can be expected to have marked reductions in seizures or be seizure-free.

## C. Temporal lobe surgery

1. Appropriate for temporal lobe seizures. This involves resection of the anterior temporal lobe.

2. Candidates demonstrate complex partial seizures with a unilateral, anterior temporal lobe focus. Recently, selective amygdalohippocampectomy has been proposed for patients with a focus in the mesial temporal region.

3. **Complications** include subtle recent memory deficits (spatial information for right-sided resections and verbal information for left-sided resections).

4. **Outcome.** Sixty to seventy percent of appropriately selected patients are ultimately seizure-free and 10% have marked reductions in seizure activity. About half of patients who become seizure-free can be expected to be weaned entirely from anticonvulsants.

## D. Frontal lobectomy

1. Resection of the frontal lobe.

2. Candidates have seizures originating from the frontal lobe.

3. **Complications.** Loss of smell on the operative side due to sacrifice of the olfactory bulb.

4. **Outcome.** Fifty-five percent of appropriately selected patients have markedly reduced seizures or are seizure-free following frontal lobectomy.

## E. Corpus callosotomy

1. Functions by preventing the interhemispheric propagation of seizures.
2. **Indications.** Drop attacks, mixed seizure disorders, life-threatening primarily or secondarily generalized seizures.
3. May be done in one or two stages. When performed in two stages, an anterior two-thirds resection is followed by a posterior resection if seizures persist.
4. **Complications** include disconnection and mutism that are usually transient. Leg weakness can occur.
5. **Outcome** is related to seizure type, with drop attacks having the best outcome (75–100% improvement) and other types of seizures improving in the range of 50%.

# Involuntary Movement Disorders

A variety of involuntary movements occur in association with neurological disease. Described here are the types of movements that suggest an underlying neurological condition. Also included is an overview of those disorders in which the main feature is some form of involuntary movement.

## I. INVOLUNTARY MOVEMENTS
  A. **Chorea.** A rapid, irregular jerk of the extremities, face, or trunk. It may be unilateral or bilateral and often migrates. Attempts to hide the movement by including it into a voluntary movement are common. Children with chorea often have the appearance of being in constant motion and are described as "restless."
  B. **Athetosis.** A slow, writhing movement of the extremity, frequently with exaggerated posture. Often found in association with chorea and described as **choreoathetosis.**
  C. **Dystonia.** Prolonged tonic contractions of the agonist and antagonist of muscle groups or individual muscles.
  D. **Myoclonus.** Irregular, frequent, transient jerks of muscle groups or individual muscles. It may be triggered by sensory stimulation **(reflex myoclonus)** or by movement **(action myoclonus).** It may or may not be rhythmic. Action myoclonus needs to be distinguished from epileptic myoclonus.
  E. **Tremor.** An oscillating movement characterized by a constant frequency. It may be present at rest (resting tremor) or with movement (intention tremor).
  F. **Ballismus.** Violent flinging movements of the extremity.
  G. **Mirror movements.** Voluntary movements in one extremity (often the hands) are "mirrored" involuntarily by the opposite extremity.
  H. **Tics/habit spasms.** Brief, repetitive, stereotyped movements such as eye-blinking or throat-clearing. These may develop transiently following a brief illness, such as sniffing following the resolution of a cold. They tend to increase in frequency with anxiety. They are distinctive in that they can be stopped with distraction, unlike pathological movements.

## II. GILLES DE LA TOURETTE'S SYNDROME
  A. A not uncommon syndrome characterized by multiple uncontrollable tics and compulsive verbal obscenities (coprolalia).
  B. Autosomal dominant inheritance with a prevalence ranging between 0.05% and 2.50%. Among males, penetrance is nearly complete and among females, penetrance is 0.71. Males are afflicted with Tourette's syndrome 3–5 times as often as females. It rarely affects blacks. The gene is located on the long arm of chromosome 18.
  C. **Onset** is generally between the ages of 2 and 10.
  D. **Features**
     1. Recurrent, involuntary tics affecting the head, face, or other motor groups.
     2. Multiple vocal tics including grunting, barking, sneezing,

and echolalia.

**3. Copopraxia.** Involuntary performance of rude and insulting gestures.

**4.** Ability to suppress tics for minutes to hours.

**5. Neuropsychiatric disturbance.** Psychiatric disorders occur in nearly 10% of patients with Tourette's syndrome, learning disturbances in about 20%, and attention deficit disorder in 35%. Obsessive-compulsive behaviors are more common in patients with Tourette's syndrome, especially in afflicted females.

**6.** Symptoms tend to fluctuate in intensity.

**E. Diagnosis** is based primarily on clinical features. EEG is abnormal in half of afflicted children. Neuroimaging reveals no abnormalities.

**F. Treatment**

**1.** Haloperidol is the drug of choice and can cause abatement of symptoms in up to 90% of cases. Unfortunately, 10–20% of children have significant extrapyramidal side effects that limit the use of the drug.

**2.** Pimozide, a dopamine antagonist, is effective in up to 70% of cases. It is typically associated with fewer side effects than haloperidol.

**3.** Clonidine has also been demonstrated to be effective in controlling the behavioral disturbances associated with Tourette's syndrome.

**G. Prognosis.** Tourette's syndrome persists into adulthood, but symptoms tend to lessen after adolescence. Eight percent of cases have a complete remission.

**III. SYDENHAM'S CHOREA** (ST. VITUS' DANCE)

**A.** A disorder characterized by choreiform movements, emotional lability, and muscular hypotonia.

**B.** Often there is a family history of chorea or rheumatic fever, but no specific inheritance pattern is notable. Most cases of Sydenham's chorea have a history of prior streptococcal infection or acute rheumatic fever. A history of emotional trauma is elicited in a significant number of patients and may play a role in the development of chorea. There is a slightly higher incidence in females.

**C. Onset** is typically between the ages of 3 and 13.

**D. Features**

**1.** Involuntary choreiform movements that increase with stress. In some cases these affect only one side (hemichorea).

**2.** Bilateral facial movements often interpreted as "making faces."

**3.** The increased motor movements at all joints cause the child to be described as "fidgety" and "restless".

**4.** The movements impair coordination. Children are often described as "clumsy".

**5.** Speech can be affected. It may become slurred and jerky.

**6.** Swallowing and breathing can also become impaired. In severe cases, feeding tubes may become necessary.

**E. Diagnosis** is made by history and clinical features. An antecedent streptococcal infection is frequently remote (several months), but serologic evidence of prior infection is often present.

**F. Treatment.** Acutely, diazepam or phenobarbital improves the neurological symptoms. Penicillin should be administered for a minimum of 10 days to eliminate any active streptococcal infection. Thereafter, prophylactic penicillin therapy should be used as per rheumatic fever protocols.

**G. Prognosis.** Progressive improvement over several months is the rule. Two thirds of patients have recurrent episodes, but these usually occur in the first 1 to 2 years following presentation. Few patients have persistent symptomatology and, if present, it tends to be minor (tremor, incoordination).

**IV. HUNTINGTON'S CHOREA** (see Chapter 2).

**V. TARDIVE DYSKINESIA**

**A.** The development of involuntary movements in association with the use of neuroleptic medications.

**B.** This disorder has no known genetic component. It is thought to be related to hypersensitivity of dopamine receptors caused by neuroleptic medications. In some series it has been noted to occur in up to 25% of hospitalized patients on neuroleptics.

**C. Onset** is usually after the child has been on neuroleptic therapy for months or years, or after dosing is increased. Some cases of tardive dyskinesia have been seen even with low-dose therapy or at the time of therapy withdrawal.

**D. Features.** Involuntary orofacial movements (chewing, tongue protrusion, lip-smacking). Less commonly, involuntary movements of extremities are seen.

**E. Diagnosis** is made by observation of the movements and a history of neuroleptic therapy. It is important to rule out other causes of movement disorders.

**F. Treatment.** Discontinuation of the medication is associated with abatement of symptoms in most cases. If symptoms persist, clonidine can be used.

**G. Prognosis.** If symptoms persist with withdrawal of medication, the prognosis is poor.

**VI. OTHERS**

**A. Benign familial tremor** (essential tremor)

**1.** Presence of a rhythmic tremor.

**2.** Autosomal dominant.

**3. Onset** is usually during puberty, but can be noted as early as 5 years of age.

**4. Features.** A rhythmic tremor (4–8 Hz) that increases with movement and is usually absent at rest. One or both upper extremities can be affected. The tremor typically does not interfere with fine motor skills. In some cases head-nodding develops.

**5. Diagnosis** is by history and evaluation of the tremor. Other basal ganglia disorders must be excluded before making a diagnosis of familial tremor.

**6. Treatment** with propranolol if needed.

**B. Benign familial chorea**

**1.** Chorea.

**2.** Autosomal dominant inheritance.

**3. Onset** is in early childhood.

**4. Features.** Chorea may be the only symptom. Other children have associated athetosis, intention tremor, hypotonia, and dysarthria.

5. **Diagnosis** is based on a positive family history and the absence of other causes of chorea.

6. **Treatment** with haloperidol is often effective.

7. **Prognosis** is good, although symptoms typically continue into adulthood.

C. **Lance-Adams syndrome** (posthypoxic myoclonus). Myoclonus developing after an episode of hypoxia. Myoclonic jerking of the extremities and facial and pharyngeal muscles typically presents shortly after the hypoxic spell and persists. Treatment with clonazepam or valproic acid is often effective.

D. **Torticollis**

1. Rotation of the head caused by a unilateral spasmodic contraction of the neck muscles, primarily the sternocleidomastoid musculature. It can be **nonfixed** (the neck is readily moved back into neutral position) or **fixed** (the neck cannot be moved into neutral position).

2. Torticollis can be a manifestation of a number of underlying disorders.

   a. Posterior fossa tumors with head tilt.

   b. Ophthalmoplegia (fourth nerve palsy) related to an underlying disorder.

   c. Cervicomedullary malformations.

   d. Cervical cord pathology (tumor, syrinx).

   e. Juvenile rheumatoid arthritis.

   f. Sternocleidomastoid injury.

   g. Intrauterine positional deformities.

3. **Benign paroxysmal torticollis** is a migraine variant with unfixed torticollis. A positive family history for migraine and transient (hours to days), unfixed torticollis in very young children suggest this diagnosis. Associated symptoms of nausea, vomiting, pallor, and irritability may be present.

4. **Sandifer syndrome** is the association of torticollis and a hiatal hernia. Gastrointestinal symptoms (nausea, vomiting, dysphagia) are common.

5. **Treatment** of the underlying precipitating factor is critical. If no specific underlying cause is found, torticollis can persist into adulthood.

# Spasticity

Spasticity is a common manifestation of neurological disease. The etiology and terminology of spasticity are described in this chapter along with a review of the pathophysiology and management options.

## I. ETIOLOGY
### A. Cerebral palsy
1. A group of disorders in which the etiologic insult occurs in the antenatal, perinatal, or early childhood period, resulting in sustained brain damage with retardation of motor development. The insult in CP is not progressive, although the manifestations of CP change with the development of the child.
2. Clinically these children have retardation of motor development involving one or all limbs and retention of primitive reflexes. Because of this they develop abnormal patterns of posture, movement, and coordination.
3. The most common cause of CP is prematurity. Other etiologies include anoxia, physical injury, kernicterus, infection, and genetic abnormalities.
4. The incidence of CP is 2.0–2.5:1000 school-age children.
5. There are four basic types of CP that are manifested in varying degrees of severity.
   a. Spastic.
   b. Dyskinetic (athetosis and others).
   c. Ataxic.
   d. Mixed (elements of spastic, dyskinetic, and ataxic forms).
6. The spastic form (75% of cases) has a number of associated descriptive terms.
   a. **Spastic quadriplegia.** Involvement of all four limbs.
   b. **Spastic diplegia.** Lower extremity involvement is more extensive than upper extremity involvement.
   c. **Spastic hemiplegia.** Involvement of one side of the body.
   d. **Spastic paraplegia.** Only lower extremity involvement (rare).
   e. **Tetraparesis.** Involvement of three limbs.
   f. **Spastic monoplegia.** Involvement of a single limb, usually an arm.
7. **Athetosis** is characterized by fluctuating tone with the body in nearly constant motion. The head is rarely in the midline. Varying degrees of athetosis occur; for example, a single hand may show athetosis.
### B. Spinal cord injury
### C. Cerebral trauma or stroke
## II. PATHOPHYSIOLOGY
A. Spasticity is an exaggerated reflex reaction with stretch of a muscle. Clinically this is manifested by hyperreflexia, clonus, and resistance to passive movement.
B. The forms of spasticity associated with CP, SCI, cerebral injury, and stroke are more complex entities and do not

represent simple spasticity. These forms of spasticity also exhibit a loss of balance between the descending inhibitory motor tracts and the excitatory anterior horn cells.

## III. TREATMENT

- **A.** Physical therapy helps prevent the development of contractures, improves mobility and function, and maximizes potential.
- **B.** Orthopedic procedures (arthodesis, osteotomies, tenotomies) treat contractures.
- **C.** Pharmacologic treatment with baclofen, dantrolene sodium, and diazepam improves spasticity in some cases.
- **D. Selective posterior rhizotomy** is the selective sectioning of abnormal posterior rootlets for the treatment of spasticity. It is primarily used in the treatment of CP, although other applications have been described (MS, SCI).
    1. SPR is beneficial in selected patients. Poor prognostic indicators include athetosis, fluctuating tone, the persistence of primary reflexes, and patient age over 17 years. Good prognostic indicators are pure spastic diplegia, no or minimal prior orthopedic intervention, intelligence, and younger age.
    2. Early operation is optimal. The abnormal activity associated with CP interferes with the development of normal motor and postural patterns. Similarly, it encourages the development of abnormal patterns. Early operation helps interrupt this cycle and maximizes the potential for the development of more normal motor patterns.
    3. With careful preoperative screening, 80% of patients can be expected to have good to excellent results from SPR.
- **E. Bilateral dorsal rhizotomy** (C1–C3) is used in the treatment of tonic neck reflexes with improvement in spasticity and upper extremity function. If extended to include C4, C5, and C6, 50% of patients will have significant respiratory problems.

# Infections

A wide variety of infectious processes affecting the nervous system occur in the pediatric patient. The accurate diagnosis of these conditions is imperative to prevent devastating damage to the developing CNS. Infections may develop in utero, during delivery, or postnatally. The timing of infection is helpful in determining a diagnosis, as certain infections are age-related.

## I. TORCH SYNDROME

    **A.** Stands for **T**oxoplasmosis, **O**ther (syphilis), **R**ubella, **C**ytomegalovirus, and **H**erpes simplex virus. It has been suggested that this mnemonic be changed to **STARCH** to include infection with human immunodeficiency virus (AIDS).

    **B.** Except for herpes simplex (which is spread as an ascending infection or during delivery through active lesions) these infections are spread transplacentally in a hematogenous manner from an infected mother.

    **C. Toxoplasmosis**

        **1.** A protozoan infection caused by *Toxoplasma gondii*.

        **2.** Severe infection usually occurs in the first or second trimester of pregnancy. If infection develops in the third trimester it is likely to be mild or asymptomatic.

        **3.** It is the second most common congenital infection after CMV.

        **4.** The incidence varies geographically from 0.2 to 5.0 per 100 pregnancies, since the parasite is spread through the consumption of undercooked meat. In the United States 1 in 10,000 infants is born with congenital toxoplasmosis.

        **5.** The majority of infants are asymptomatic. In symptomatic infants the typical triad is ventriculomegaly, intracranial calcifications, and chorioretinitis. Chorioretinitis is the most common finding. Other systemic effects include hyperbilirubinemia, hepatosplenomegaly, and anemia.

        **6.** CNS manifestations include seizures, diffuse intracranial calcifications, ventriculomegaly (20–50%), microcephaly (15%), neuronal migration anomalies, infarction, and meningoencephalitis.

        **7. Diagnosis**

            **a.** Isolation of the organism from blood, CSF, or the placenta.

            **b.** **Sabin-Feldman dye test** has been mostly replaced by the IgG indirect immunofluorescent antibody test.

            **c.** **IgM fluorescent antibody** measures fetal IgM antibodies.

        **8. Radiographic features**

            **a.** **Skull x-rays.** Diffuse calcification.

            **b.** **CT.** Diffuse and periventricular calcifications, basal ganglia calcification, and hydrocephalus secondary to aqueductal stenosis.

            **c.** **MRI.** Migrational anomalies, pachygyria, and demyelination in older patients.

**9. Treatment**

   **a.** Hydrocephalus associated with toxoplasmosis is caused by the inflammatory reaction within the meninges and vascular involvement with the parasite causing thrombosis of the ependymal vessels. Hydrocephalus is considered a progressive disease and should be shunted. Ventriculomegaly is secondary to atrophy (non-progressive) and must be distinguished.

   **b.** Sulfadiazine 50–100 mg/kg/24h PO divided bid and pyrimethamine 1 mg/kg/24h PO divided bid for 30 days, followed by spiramycin 100 mg/kg/24h PO divided q12h (available from the Centers for Disease Control with guidelines for use). Supplemental folic acid 1 mg/kg/24h IM should be administered because pyrimethamine is a folic acid antagonist. Steroid use remains controversial.

**10. Prognosis** is related to the severity and extent of disease. The presence of significant neurological symptoms portends a poor prognosis, with < 10% being normal. With significant systemic symptoms, < 20% will be normal. Mental retardation, seizures, spasticity, and severe visual impairment are the usual sequelae.

**D. Syphilis**

   **1.** Infection with the spirochete *Treponema pallidum*.

   **2.** Transplacental spread of the organism usually in the second or third trimester. If the mother has untreated primary, or secondary syphilis, the risk to the fetus is increased. With a maternal infection late in gestation there is a decreased incidence of congenital syphilis.

   **3.** The incidence has decreased with the availability of penicillin, but cases persist.

   **4.** Congenital syphilis is usually asymptomatic until after the second week of life. Features include rashes (vesiculobullous or papulosquamous), mucocutaneous lesions, hepatosplenomegaly, lymphadenopathy, anemia, hyperbilirubinemia, osteochondritis of the distal metaphysis, and periostitis.

   **5. CNS features.** Meningitis, hydrocephalus, ventriculomegaly, seizures, cranial nerve palsies, (usually VII, but also III, IV, or VI), infarctions with focal deficits, and signs and symptoms of increased ICP.

   **6. Diagnosis**

   **a.** Identification of the organism in placental, cutaneous, or mucocutaneous lesions using dark-field microscopy.

   **b.** VDRL test (nontreponemal, nonspecific assay) of serum or CSF for the presence of antibodies. High false-positive rate.

   **c.** FTA-ABS test depends on the presence of antibodies specific to *T. pallidum*.

   **d.** FTA-ABS-IgM reacts only with IgM antibodies (fetal produced).

   **7. Treatment**

   **a. Without CNS involvement.** Penicillin G procaine 50,000 U/kg/24h IM qd for 10 days or penicillin G benzathine 50,000 U/kg IM weekly for 3 weeks.

      **b. With CNS involvement.** For children over 12, use
penicillin G procaine 2.4 million U IM qd for 10 days. For
children ages 2–11, use penicillin G benzathine 2.4 U IM
weekly for 3 weeks. For neonates and children less than
2 years of age, administer penicillin G benzathine 50,000
U/kg IM as a single dose.

**E. Rubella**
  1. Infection with the rubella virus.
  2. Transplacental transfer during the first trimester. The
transfer of the virus causes teratogenic and destructive
effects.
  3. Low incidence with use of the rubella vaccine.
  4. Early infection is associated with ocular, cardiac, and hearing defects. Neurological deficits are most common in infections occurring in the first 8 weeks of pregnancy.
  5. Systemic presentation: stillbirth, intrauterine growth retardation, cataracts, chorioretinitis, cardiovascular anomalies, skeletal lesions.
  6. **CNS features.** Meningoencephalitis, lethargy,
opisthotonos, seizures, hypotonia, and irritability.
  7. **Diagnosis**
    **a.** Isolation of the virus from the nasopharynx, stool, urine,
or CSF.
    **b.** Serologic assay for IgM antibody.
  8. **Radiographic.** A single reported case of rubella with CT
imaging showed cerebral white matter hypodensity and
calcification of the basal ganglia.
  9. **Treatment** is supportive. The use of antiviral agents may
be considered.
 10. **Prognosis.** Sixty percent of cases display mild to severe
neurological deficits. Hearing loss may be progressive.

**F. Cytomegalovirus**
  1. Infection with CMV.
  2. Transplacental infection in the first or second trimester.
Infection may also occur at the time of birth, through breast
milk or related to a blood transfusion; however, infections
through these modes of transmission usually lack serious
neurological sequelae.
  3. The most common congenital infection in the United States,
it affects 0.2–2.2% of newborns.
  4. **Presentation.** Ninety to ninety-five percent of cases are
asymptomatic in the neonatal period. Symptoms that develop include hepatosplenomegaly, hyperbilirubinemia,
anemia, and inguinal hernias.
  5. **CNS features.** Microcephaly (up to 50%), seizures,
meningoencephalitis, and cerebral palsy usually become
apparent by 2 years of age.
  6. **Diagnosis**
    **a.** Isolation of the virus from urine, throat culture, or CSF.
Electron microscopy of viral particles is helpful.
    **b.** Persistence of IgG titers with a complement fixation test.
    **c.** IgM detection with immunofluoresence.
  7. **Radiographic**
    **a. Skull x-rays.** Periventricular calcification.

   **b. CT.** Atrophy, hydrocephalus, ventriculomegaly, periventricular and parenchymal calcification.

   **c. MRI.** Gliosis and neuronal migration anomalies.

8. **Treatment** is supportive. Antiviral agents are of questionable benefit.

9. **Prognosis** is based on the degree of infection. The presence of neurological symptoms suggests a poor outcome, with 95% of patients having seizures, mental retardation, and bilateral hearing loss. Asymptomatic patients may develop sensorineural hearing loss and have minimal intellectual impairment.

## G. Herpes simplex

1. Infection with herpes simplex virus. In congenital herpes this is usually the type 2 virus.

2. Most commonly acquired during delivery through an infected birth canal. Ascending, transplacental, and postnatal infections occur.

3. The incidence is about 30:100,000 live births.

4. Symptoms usually develop within 7 days after birth. They may be localized or systemic. Systemic manifestations include hepatomegaly, hyperbilirubinemia, bleeding, vesicular rashes, and keratoconjunctivitis.

5. CNS involvement may present with lethargy and poor feeding and progress to irritability, seizures, opisthotonos, and coma.

6. **Radiography**
   
   **a. CT.** Acutely there is a lucency of the cerebral hemispheres (focal or diffuse) primarily in the white matter. The temporal and frontal lobes may be preferentially affected. Ultimately, atrophy and encephalomalacia predominate.

   **b. MR.** Acute herpes may not be recognized in the neonate because of the lack of myelination.

7. **Diagnosis**

   **a.** Cytology on scrapings from lesions.

   **b.** Isolation of virus from lesions.

   **c.** Serologic studies are not very useful because of the passive immunity passed from the mother and the delay in IgM production by the neonate.

   **d.** Brain biopsy may be necessary.

8. **Treatment.** Neonates should be treated with vidarabine monohydrate 15–30 mg/kg IV as a single daily dose and in children 15 mg/kg/24h as a 12–24-hour infusion. Treatment should continue for 10 days. Alternatively, acyclovir therapy for 7 days can be used. In neonates, use acyclovir 30 mg/kg/24h IV divided q8h; in children, 250 mg/mm$^2$ q8h.

9. **Prognosis.** There is an 80% mortality rate with disseminated disease in the neonate. Survivors are usually significantly impaired.

# II. MENINGITIS

**A.** Meningitis can be caused by bacteria, viruses, fungi, or protozoa. It is an inflammatory process affecting predominantly the meninges.

## B. Bacterial meningitis

**1.** The incidence is 3–10:100,000 children.
  **a. Neonatal pathogens.** *Escherichia coli* and group B streptococcus.
  **b. Infancy.** *Haemophilus influenzae, Streptococcus pneumoniae, Neisseria meningitidis.*
  **c. Older children.** *S. pneumoniae, N. meningitidis.*
**2. Pathogenesis**
  **a.** Colonization of the upper respiratory tract with invasion of the nasal mucosa into the blood stream with meningeal seeding.
  **b.** Direct extension from infected sinuses, otitis media, or mastoiditis.
  **c.** Cranial osteomyelitis or a compound fracture of the skull.
  **d.** Fractures of the cribriform plate or paranasal sinuses.
  **e.** Neurocutaneous fistulae.
**3. Presentation.** Fever, irritability, lethargy, headache, meningismus, seizures, and progressive obtundation.
**4. Diagnosis**
  **a.** LP with CSF showing an elevated WBC count (predominantly PMN) and a low glucose suggests bacterial meningitis.
  **b.** Partially treated bacterial meningitis may lack PMN.
  **c.** CIE.
  **d.** CSF with an elevated WBC count (predominantly lymphocytes), elevated protein, and a low glucose suggests a tuberculous, fungal, or viral meningitis.
**5. Treatment** should be instituted rapidly based on age, CSF characteristics, and results of CIE.
  **a.** Unknown bacterial etiology in a newborn: Ampicillin or penicillin G and an aminoglycoside.
  **b.** Unknown bacterial etiology at 1–3 months of age: Ampicillin and cefotaxime.
  **c.** Unknown bacterial etiology after 3 months of age: Ampicillin and chloramphenicol or cefuroxime, cefotaxime, or ceftriaxone.
**6. Neurosurgical sequelae**
  **a.** Subdural effusions (10%). The differentiation between sterile effusions and empyema can be assessed by subdural tap or with contrasted CT. Empyemas have an enhancing membrane. Effusions rarely require surgical treatment, but when they do, continuous subdural drainage or a subdural to peritoneal shunt may be required.
  **b.** Ventriculomegaly may be related to atrophy from the destructive effects of the organism on the brain. In some cases it may be progressive and associated with increased pressure necessitating shunt placement.
**C. Viral meningitis**
  **1.** Most commonly caused by enterovirus.
  **2.** Tends to be seasonal, with an increased incidence in summer and fall.
  **3.** Epidemics of viral meningitis occur.
  **4.** Presentation is with fever, malaise, headache, neck pain, and photophobia.

**5.** CSF studies may show a mild pleocytosis, initially with predominantly neutrophils and then mononuclear cells. The protein may be slightly increased and the glucose normal to mildly depressed.

**6.** The duration of illness is 1–2 weeks with complete recovery as the rule.

## D. Aseptic meningitis

**1.** An inflammatory process of the meninges with CSF pleocytosis (initially leukocytes and later mononuclear cells), frequently normal to slightly increased protein, and a normal glucose.

**2.** Aseptic meningitis may occur after craniotomy for brain tumor.

**3.** The term aseptic is a misnomer, since infection may be present. A variety of diseases and infections have been associated with aseptic meningitis syndrome. These include the following.

   **a.** Viruses.

   **b.** Lyme disease (*Borrelia burgdorferi*).

   **c.** Fungal infections.

   **d.** Malignancy (leukemia, brain tumors).

   **e.** Vasculitic disorders.

   **f.** Kawasaki disease.

   **g.** Partially treated bacterial meningitis.

   **h.** Mycobacterium tuberculosis, atypical mycobacterium.

   **i.** Parasitic infections.

**4. Presentation.** Headache, nuchal rigidity, and photophobia with the above CSF findings.

**5.** Infection must be searched for and ruled out.

**6. Treatment** is primarily supportive if no source of infection is found.

## E. Tuberculous meningitis

**1.** Infection with *Mycobacterium tuberculosis*.

**2.** Tuberculous meningitis develops within 3–6 months of the primary infection.

**3.** The mechanism of spread is hematogenous, usually from a pulmonary focus.

**4. Presentation** is generally insidious with irritability, lethargy, and a low-grade fever. Progression to declining consciousness, seizures, and signs and symptoms of increased ICP follow, usually within several days to 2 weeks.

**5.** CSF

   **a.** Protein may be normal initially and then rise to high levels.

   **b.** A predominance of lymphocytes or PMN.

   **c.** Glucose is normal initially and then declines to very low levels.

   **d.** Culture of the organism is very difficult and all sources should be sought (CSF, gastric aspiration, sputum) in addition to placement of a TB skin test. All cultures must be kept for a minimum of 6 weeks.

**6. Treatment**

   **a.** Isoniazid, rifampin, and pyrazinamide (liver function tests [LFTs] must be monitored). Streptomycin, ethambutol, or ethionamide can be added if resistant organisms are isolated.

 b. Increased ICP may necessitate placement of a ventriculostomy. Shunt placement may become necessary for progressive hydrocephalus.

III. **ENCEPHALITIS** is an inflammatory process affecting the brain and often the meninges. For this reason these conditions are often referred to as **meningoencephalitis**. It can be of viral, bacterial, or parasitic origin. Most cases of encephalitis present with an altered level of consciousness, lethargy, meningismus, seizures, spasticity, and weakness. CSF is useful in confirming a diagnosis of encephalitis. LP must be performed with caution because of the risk of increased ICP. Therapy is available for most bacterial and protozoal infections. Viral encephalitis is generally treated with supportive measures.

A. **Arboviral encephalitis.** These viruses are spread by arthropods (ticks, mosquitoes).

 1. **St. Louis encephalitis**

   a. **Epidemiology.** Epidemic in the Atlantic states and in the Mississippi valley. Endemic in the western United States. Most cases present in late summer or early fall. Under the age of 9, the attack rate (for the virus) is 4.3: 100,000.

   b. **Features.** Half of infected children develop a fairly benign syndrome of viral meningitis. The other half present with a severe encephalitis. Often the antecedent infection is mild or asymptomatic.

   c. **Diagnosis.** CSF findings are consistent with a viral encephalitis (lymphocytic pleocytosis, elevated protein, and normal glucose). A minimum of a fourfold elevation in antibody titers between the acute and convalescent sera is diagnostic. Pathological findings include a diffuse vascular congestion and edema in the perivascular spaces and throughout the meninges.

   d. **Course.** Symptoms are usually apparent for 1 to 2 weeks.

   e. **Treatment** is supportive. No vaccine is currently available.

   f. **Prognosis** is better in children than adults. The mortality rate is as high as 22%. Significant neurological sequelae persist in up to 10% of cases and include change in personality, gait impairment, visual impairment, and speech difficulties.

 2. **Western equine encephalitis**

   a. **Epidemiology.** Occurs in the western United States as a result of infection with a group A arbovirus. Horses with encephalitis appear to be the source of this virus, which is then transmitted by mosquitoes. Up to 30% of cases affect infants.

   b. **Features.** Infants present with irritability, fever, meningismus, seizures, and a bulging fontanelle. Older children often have a history of a flulike illness prior to developing symptoms of encephalitis.

   c. **Diagnosis.** CSF findings consistent with encephalitis

and a minimum fourfold elevation in antibodies between the acute and convalescent sera.

**d. Course.** Symptoms last about 10 days. Fatal cases have a much more rapid evolution.

**e. Treatment** is supportive. No vaccination is available.

**f. Prognosis.** The mortality rate ranges from 10–30%. Permanent deficits are common. The younger the child, the greater the long-term sequelae. At least half of infected infants have persistent seizures, developmental retardation, microcephaly, or motor impairment. Parkinsonism is a late finding in many afflicted patients. This is probably related to the significant pathological changes noted in the substantia nigra on autopsy studies.

### 3. Eastern equine encephalitis

**a. Epidemiology.** This uncommon form of encephalitis occurs along the eastern seaboard, predominantly in the mid-Atlantic states.

**b. Features.** Onset is abrupt with vomiting, high fever, meningismus, altered consciousness, and seizures.

**c. Diagnosis.** CSF demonstrates an elevated WBC count (250–2000 cells/$\mu$l) that is almost exclusively polymorphonuclear cells. This progresses to a predominantly mononuclear proliferation within 3 days. A fourfold increase in antibody titers between acute and convalescent titers confirms the diagnosis.

**d. Course.** A fulminant course with symptoms progressing in 48 hours.

**e. Treatment** is supportive; no vaccine is available.

**f. Prognosis.** The mortality rate is significant (up to 65%). Sixty percent of survivors have significant sequelae including seizures, mental retardation, deafness, and motor impairment.

## IV. INFECTIONS OF THE SPINAL CORD

### A. Transverse myelitis

1. A rapidly progressive weakness in the lower extremities with sphincter dysfunction and loss of sensation.

2. **Etiology.** Transverse myelitis is often preceded by a viral illness and is thought to be related to a viral-induced cell-mediated autoimmune response. It has been proposed that an autoimmune-induced vasculitis results in an inadequate blood supply to the spinal cord.

3. **Pathology.** Changes can be transverse (extending over several spinal segments). The spinal cord is significantly necrotic, with a cellular infiltrate replacing most of the nervous elements.

4. **Features**

   **a.** An antecedent viral infection is reported in over half of cases.

   **b.** Sensory loss in the extremities, back, or abdomen. A thoracic sensory level is most commonly found, but impairment to cervical and lumbar levels is also reported. Proprioception and vibration remain intact.

   **c.** Rectal tone is markedly decreased.

**d.** A rapidly progressive paraparesis. The upper extremities are rarely involved.

**e.** Hypotonia followed by hypertonia.

**f. Devic's disease.** Transverse myelitis in association with optic neuritis.

5. **Diagnosis** is based on clinical history, examination, and exclusion of other causes of acute paraparesis (GBS, MS, spinal cord tumor). CSF often has an elevated protein level and pleocytosis.

6. **Course.** Symptoms evolve rapidly, with the peak deficit presenting within 3 days of onset. Symptoms persist for months, with return of function usually beginning within 1 month from the onset of symptoms.

7. **Treatment** with steroids has not been demonstrated to have any significant effect on outcome. However, steroids continue to be administered in many institutions.

8. **Prognosis.** Complete recovery within 6 months is the rule. However, some children will remain significantly impaired and require wheelchairs for mobility.

**B. Poliomyelitis**

1. An acute infectious disorder caused by one of three polioviruses (enteroviruses). Due to widespread immunization programs, infection with poliovirus is infrequent.

2. **Etiology and pathology.** The poliovirus affects the motor neurons of the CNS. The anterior horn cells of the spinal cord are predominantly affected. Within the brain, layers 3 and 5 of the precentral gyrus, the thalamus, globus pallidus, cerebellar vermis, and deep cerebellar nuclei are affected.

3. **Features.** The illness is biphasic, with a minor phase corresponding to the period of viremia and the major illness following.

    **a. Minor illness.** Fever, sore throat, myalgias, headache, and gastrointestinal disturbance.

    **b. Major illness** follows the minor illness after 2–3 asymptomatic days. It is characterized by meningismus, fever, severe myalgias, headache, and vomiting. This may or may not progress to paralysis.

    **c. Paralytic stage.** This usually develops within 1–2 days of the onset of the major illness. Pain (in particular back pain), lethargy, irritability, and paralysis progress over hours to days. The paralysis is flaccid and asymmetric, although the legs are most commonly involved. Autonomic dysfunction is not uncommon.

    **d. Bulbar poliomyelitis** involves the ocular, pharyngeal, and facial musculature. Pulmonary edema, respiratory compromise, cardiac arrhythmias, and hypertension are commonly noted.

4. **Diagnosis.** History and clinical examination. CSF demonstrates an elevated WBC count. Initially this is predominantly polymorphonuclear cells, and then it is mostly mononuclear cells. The protein may not be elevated until well into the illness. CSF glucose is normal. The virus can be isolated from stool or the oropharynx.

5. **Course.** The incubation period is between 3 and 35 days

(mean, 17 days). The minor illness phase lasts 24 to 48 hours. In approximately 8% of cases no further symptoms develop. In 1–2% of cases, there is a 2- to 5-day asymptomatic period followed by progression to a major illness and paralytic polio. Recovery of motor function typically begins within several weeks of the onset of paralysis. Some recovery can be expected through the first year following illness.

6. **Treatment** is primarily prevention through widespread vaccination programs of an orally administered live attenuated virus vaccine or an inactivated poliomyelitis vaccine. If polio develops because of failure to receive vaccination or, in rare cases, in response to vaccination with the live attenuated vaccine, treatment is supportive.

7. **Prognosis.** The mortality associated with polio is about 5%. Severely paralyzed muscles become normal in 20% of cases and regain some function in half of cases. Moderately paralyzed muscles recover to normal or nearly so in 90% of cases. Recurrent episodes are rare.

## V. CYSTICERCOSIS

A. Parasitic infection caused by ingestion of the eggs of the larval pork tapeworm *Taenia solium*.

B. **Pathogenesis.** Once ingested, the embryo is freed from the egg and invades the blood supply within the gastrointestinal tract to be spread hematogenously to the CNS, skeletal muscles, eyes, and other organs. Once deposited, they develop into cysticerci (larvae) and remain there.

C. This disease is endemic in certain geographical areas (Mexico, Central America, South America, Asia, South Africa, and India). In large part due to immigration, cysticercosis has become a fairly common entity in the United States, particularly the Southwest.

D. CNS involvement is common (60–90% of cases). Cysticerci occur intracranially (parenchymal, intraventricular, meningeal) and intraspinally. Intraspinal lesions are rare in children.

E. **Pathology.** The presence of cysticercus in the nervous system elicits an immune response of variable intensity. It is often the inflammatory response that produces the symptoms. Vasculitis is typically present in the area of infection. Infection can be solitary or multiple (up to several hundred).

F. **Presentation** is highly variable, and depends on where the lesions are located. A high index of suspicion in patients at risk is important in making the diagnosis. Fifty percent of cases will present with seizures. Cysticercosis is the most common cause of seizures in some parts of the world. Other cases present with increased ICP, basal arachnoiditis, and focal neurological deficits. Children, in particular, are prone to develop cerebral edema with parenchymal lesions.

G. **Radiology**
  1. **Brain parenchymal lesions** (most common site).
     a. **Vesicular stage.** Lesions 3–12 months old, at which time the cysticercus is fully-grown. The fully grown larva with a bladder is surrounded by a thin capsule without an inflammatory reaction. On imaging studies these appear

as round cysts with a mural nodule (the head of the larva, or scolex). The fluid follows the appearance of CSF on CT and MRI. The scolex is 1–2 mm in size and isointense to the brain. Typically the lesions occur at the gray-white junction and are more often multiple, though single lesions occur.

  **b. Colloidal vesicular stage.** Twelve to eighteen months after infection, the larva dies and begins to degenerate, inciting an inflammatory response. On imaging this is distinguished by the development of a cyst wall that enhances, surrounding edema, and an increased signal intensity within the cyst.

  **c. Third stage (calcification).** The contents of the cyst become calcified, and the inflammatory cyst wall thickens and appears granulomatous. On MRI T1-weighted images, the lesions enhance and are isointense to the brain; on T2-weighted images they are hypointense to isointense. CT is particularly useful for demonstrating calcification within these lesions.

**2. Intraventricular lesions**

  **a.** Seven to twenty percent of cases of intracranial cysticercosis have intraventricular lesions. The fourth ventricle is the most common site.

  **b.** CT may suggest enlargement of the fourth ventricle.

  **c.** MRI is the study of choice because it may demonstrate intraventricular lesions.

**3. Cisternal lesions**

  **a.** Caused by *Cysticercus racemosus* (clustered larva without a scolex) or *Cysticercus cellulosae* (larva with a scolex and bladder).

  **b.** Cisternal infection by *C. cellulosae* is difficult to identify. The cisterns may demonstrate a subtle focal widening on CT or MRI.

  **c.** *C. racemosus* may occupy the cisterns and appear as a several-centimeter lesion of CSF density. This form tends to occur in the basal cisterns and cause a basal arachnoiditis that enhances on MRI or CT.

**4.** Intraspinal lesions are rare. They may be intramedullary or in the subarachnoid space. CT or myelography may be necessary to image subarachnoid cysts. MRI is useful for imaging intramedullary cysts that have an appearance similar to those in the brain.

**H. Diagnosis**

  **1.** High-risk populations are diagnosed with radiographic images.

  **2.** CSF with increased cells or protein. The combination of a complement fixation test and ELISA for cysticercus antigens within the CSF can accurately diagnose **active** neurocysticercosis in 95% of cases. Parenchymal cysticercosis is more likely to have normal CSF.

  **3.** Serum and CSF IgG antibodies to cysticercus antigens can also be assayed.

**I. Treatment**

  **1.** Praziquantel 20 mg/kg/24h divided q8h for 14 days may be used. Steroids should be started 2–3 days prior to the initiation of praziquantel in neurocysticercosis.

2. **Surgical intervention.** In general, if the diagnosis is known, surgery is not necessary except in the following circumstances.

   **a. Hydrocephalus.** Lesions causing an obstructive hydrocephalus may be removed, if possible, or shunt placement may be necessary.

   **b. Seizures.** Lesions that are surgically accessible and are a source of focal seizures should be considered for surgical treatment.

   **c. Large cysts** (racemose cysticercosis) may cause mass effect or compressive symptoms and require surgical intervention.

## VI. SUPPURATIVE INFECTIONS

### A. Cranial

1. **Scalp infections** are seen rarely, in large part because of the vascularity of the scalp. However, scalp infections complicating traumatic lacerations and surgical incisions and from intrauterine fetal scalp monitoring occur. Debridement and 7 to 10 days of antibiotics for all but the most minor cases are usually adequate therapy.

2. **Osteomyelitis of the cranial vault**

   **a.** Usually occurs as a consequence of a compound skull fracture from trauma or as a complication of surgery. Other etiologies include direct extension from an infected sinus or otitis media; secondary to the use of fetal scalp monitors in utero; or at the pin sites from halo placement.

   **b. Presentation.** Fever, local erythema, swelling, and tenderness are the usual presenting signs and symptoms. The peripheral WBC count may be elevated. Early osteomyelitis can be demonstrated using radionuclide bone scans. Plain x-rays will begin to suggest osteomyelitis within 2 weeks of the infection. Initially the affected bone will appear "moth-eaten."

   **c. Treatment** is with intravenous antibiotics for at least 2 weeks, followed by up to 12 weeks of oral antibiotics. There is a risk of the development of an epidural abscess whenever osteomyelitis of the skull is present. If infection occurs after craniotomy, it may be necessary to remove the bone flap.

3. **Epidural abscess.** Usually develops as an extension of infection from the sinuses, mastoid air cells, or skull. They are often small and symptomatic only as infection. These cases may be amenable to medical treatment alone. If they enlarge, they may cause pressure and be symptomatic as mass lesions. Then treatment is surgical, followed by intravenous antibiotics for 2 weeks.

4. **Subdural empyemas** usually develop secondary to other infectious processes (sinusitis, otitis media, osteomyelitis) or as a result of the hematogenous infection of a subdural hematoma or an effusion associated with meningitis. Symptoms of an infectious process (elevated WBC count, fever) are common. Signs and symptoms of increased ICP and

focal deficits may develop as the empyema enlarges. Treatment is drainage followed by intravenous antibiotics for 2 weeks.

5. **Brain abscess**
   a. Develops through a variety of mechanisms: direct extension (from sinusitis, otitis media, mastoiditis); hematogenous spread (usually in association with congenital heart disease); secondary to penetrating trauma; through infection of a dermal sinus tract; or within a dermoid tumor.
   b. With current widespread and early use of antibiotics in the treatment of infections, and early surgical correction of congenital heart disease, brain abscesses are seen infrequently in children.
   c. Presentation in infants is typically increased ICP (full fontanelle, irritability, and lethargy) without fever. Older children present with fever, irritability, focal neurological symptoms, and seizures (50%).
   d. Once an organism invades the parenchyma, the acute cerebritis phase begins, which lasts 4–5 days. During this phase a vascular response occurs with polymorphonuclear cells attacking the bacteria and causing edema. Microscopic hemorrhage occurs during the acute phase. At the end of the first week, the late phase of cerebritis begins with a central area of necrosis developing and granulation tissue forming. At the end of the second week, a capsule begins to form and mature into a three-layered structure—an inner layer of granulation tissue, a middle collagenous layer, and an outer gliotic layer.
   e. Imaging studies depend on the age of infection. Ultimately, these are imaged on CT (+/-C) and MRI (+/-G) as hypodense lesions with ring enhancement. Surrounding edema is common.
   f. Medical treatment is usually effective. Frequently, surgery is required for diagnosis, to drain the lesion, to culture the organism, or because of a deterioration in neurological status.

B. **Spinal**
   1. **Congenital dermal sinus tracts** communicate with the neural elements. If they become infected they can cause CNS infection.
   2. **Spondylitis** is rarely seen in children. The two most common organisms are tuberculosis and *Staphylococcus aureus*. Unless infection extends into the epidural space and causes cord compression, surgery is not indicated.
   3. **Discitis** is an inflammation of the disc space most commonly found in the lumbar region. The etiology is thought to be hematogenous spread of infection through the rich vascular network supplying the disc in children. In children, organisms are rarely cultured from the blood or disc space, but when they are, *S. aureus* is found most commonly. Presentation is with persistent back or leg pain. Plain films may show narrowing of the disk space. CT can demonstrate demineralization of the end plate initially, and

later, frank erosion. MRI T2-weighted images show loss of disc space height, flattening of the center of the disc, and a decreased signal within the disc. Treatment is bedrest. Antibiotics have been associated with a somewhat shorter course.

4. **Epidural abscess** is rarely seen in children. The etiology is hematogenous spread of infection. Presentation is variable, but usually fever, irritability, lower extremity weakness, and pain are noted. CT (+/-C) or MRI (+/-G) will readily demonstrate these lesions. Treatment is surgical when compression is present. Without compression, aggressive medical treatment can be effective.

5. **Spinal cord abscess** is rarely seen. It may arise as a result of hematogenous spread of an organism or through a dermal sinus. Presentation typically is with evidence of the primary infection, back pain, and meningismus. CT (+/-C) and MRI (+/-G) demonstrate these lesions readily. Treatment is surgical.

## VII. HUMAN IMMUNODEFICIENCY VIRUS (HIV)

A. In 1989 there were 1681 cases of pediatric AIDS. Thirteen percent were acquired from contaminated blood products, 78% were perinatally acquired, and 6% were acquired through the treatment of hemophilia or other coagulopathies.

B. In 1991 there were an estimated 10,000–20,000 HIV-positive children.

C. HIV is an RNA virus that infects and disables the immune system, causing B- and T-cell dysfunction.

D. **Clinical manifestations**
   1. Failure to thrive.
   2. Lymphadenopathy.
   3. Hepatosplenomegaly.
   4. Chronic diarrhea.
   5. Chronic thrush.
   6. Interstitial pulmonary disease.
   7. Recurrent bacterial infections.
   8. Opportunistic infections (*Pneumocystis carinii* pneumonia, disseminated candidiasis, *Mycobacterium avium–intracellulare*, disseminated ulcerative herpes simplex, and Toxoplasmosis).

E. **CNS manifestations**
   1. Developmental delays.
   2. Cognitive impairment.
   3. Acquired microcephaly.
   4. Corticospinal tract dysfunction.
   5. Myelopathy.
   6. Peripheral neuropathy.
   7. CNS lymphoma.
   8. Strokes/infarctions.
   9. Intracerebral hemorrhage.

F. **CT.** Cerebral atrophy with ventriculomegaly, attenuation of white matter, and calcification of the basal ganglia.

G. **Treatment**
   1. Treatment of opportunistic infections.
   2. AZT.

**3.**Interferon.

**4.**IV gamma globulins.

**H. Prognosis.** Currently there is no effective cure for HIV infection.

## VIII. LYME DISEASE

**A.** A multisystem disorder resulting from the bite of a tick (*Ixodes dammini*) with transmission of the spirochete *B. burgdorferi*.

**B. General features**

**1.**Skin rash. An erythematous macular lesion that begins locally and may spread. It typically appears within 4–20 days after the tick bite and resolves within 3 weeks.

**2.**Myalgias, arthralgias, headache, fever.

**3.**Cardiac abnormalities. Conduction abnormalities, myocarditis, pericarditis.

**C. Neurological features** typically present within 1–3 months following infection. The symptoms vary, but can include any of the following features:

**1.**Aseptic meningitis.

**2.**Meningoencephalitis.

**3.**Cranial neuropathies, most commonly of the seventh and eighth nerves.

**4.**Paralysis (spastic or flaccid).

**5.**Cerebellar dysfunction.

**6.**Seizures.

**7.**Radiculoneuritis.

**D. Diagnosis**

**1.**Serologic diagnosis (elevated IgG and IgM antibodies to *B. burgdorferi*) is helpful; however, seronegative cases of Lyme disease have been reported.

**2.**The organism can sometimes be isolated from skin, CSF, or serum.

**3.**MRI demonstrates punctate hyperintensities on T1- and T2-weighted images in the cerebral hemisphere white matter.

**E. Treatment**

**1.**In most cases tetracycline (25–50 mg/kg/24h PO divided bid to qid) is the drug of choice for children over age 8.

**2.**Young children and patients with significant meningoencephalitic symptoms should be treated with IV penicillin V (50 mg/kg/24h in divided doses with a minimum of 1 g/24h and a maximum of 2 g/24h) for 10–20 days.

**F. Prognosis** is variable.

# Metabolic Abnormalities

This chapter covers a variety of relatively rare disorders characterized by abnormalities in one or more metabolic pathways, resulting in functional impairment or frank disease. The CNS is affected by many of these disorders. The majority of metabolic disorders are inherited through autosomal recessive transmission. Parents of children with metabolic disorders will benefit from genetic counseling, as will the children themselves. Prenatal diagnosis for high-risk parents can be accomplished through amniocentesis or chorionic villus biopsy in some cases. With diagnosis comes the potential for treatment. Medications, replacement therapy or dietary restrictions, and dietary supplements can be effective in some cases.

## I. DISORDERS OF AMINO ACID (AA) METABOLISM
### A. Phenylketonuria
1. Results from the absence of **phenylalanine hydroxylase** with failure to convert phenylalanine to tyrosine. This is the most common disorder of AA metabolism.
2. Autosomal recessive transmission. Rare in people of Jewish or African descent. The carrier rate is about 1 in 50 Caucasians. The frequency ranges from 1:4000 live births in Northern Ireland to 1:12,000 live births in the northeastern United States.
3. Normal at birth with progressive developmental delay over the first 12 months of life, progressing to mental retardation if left untreated.
4. **Features**
   a. Fair hair and skin.
   b. Eczema.
   c. Irritability.
   d. "Mousy" urine odor.
5. **Diagnosis**
   a. Increased serum phenylalanine.
   b. Decreased serum tyrosine.
   c. Abnormal urinary metabolites found are phenylpyruvic acid and o-hydroxyphenylacetic acid.
6. Though screening is common at birth, 10% of children with PKU will not be diagnosed because it takes time for the increase in PKU to reach the threshold level of the assay.
7. Treatment is the dietary restriction of phenylalanine intake combined with tyrosine supplementation.
8. **Maternal PKU** refers to a pregnant woman with PKU whose child develops symptoms of PKU that cause in utero damage to the fetal brain without the fetus sharing the metabolic disorder. Mental retardation occurs in 90% of infants affected by maternal PKU.

### B. Homocystinuria
1. Increased levels of plasma and urinary homocystine caused by three separate metabolic defects.
   a. **Cystathionine synthase deficiency (classical form).** Increased homocystine, homocysteine, and methionine

in blood, and urine with decreased cystathionine. Children are usually mentally retarded. Treatment is a diet low in methionine and supplementation with pyridoxine.

**b. Methyltetrahydrofolate methyltransferase deficiency.** Increased serum homocystine and homocysteine with decreased methionine. Treatment is vitamin $B_{12}$ supplementation.

**c. 5,10-methylene-tetrahydrofolate reductase deficiency.** Normal or decreased serum methionine. Children have myopathy, behavioral disturbances, and psychotic episodes. Treatment with folic acid.

2. Autosomal recessive transmission.

3. **Features** (involvement of the skeletal system, eye, CNS, and vascular system)

   **a.** Marfanoid habitus.

   **b.** Dislocated lenses (develops between 3 and 10 years of age).

   **c.** Arachnodactyly (less than 50%).

   **d.** Recurrent thromboembolism.

   **e.** Mental retardation.

## C. Nonketotic hyperglycemia

1. Increased glycine in blood, urine, and CSF.

2. Presents in neonates with spasticity, seizures, and growth retardation.

3. **Treatment.** Low-protein diet and sodium benzoate administration.

4. Regardless of treatment, these children are severely neurologically impaired. Many cases are fatal.

## D. Maple syrup urine disorder

1. Increased levels of branched-chain keto acid metabolites resulting from a defect in decarboxylation of the branched-chain AA (isoleucine, leucine, valine).

2. **Clinical presentation**

   **a.** Urine with the odor of maple syrup.

   **b.** Seizures.

   **c.** Spasticity.

   **d.** Respiratory irregularities.

   **e.** Mental retardation.

3. **Treatment.** Limited intake of branched-chain AA, which is very difficult to sustain.

## E. Isovaleric aciduria

1. Inability to decarboxylate leucine.

2. **Presentation.** Intermittent but recurrent acute episodes of acidosis, vomiting, coma, anemia, leukopenia, and thrombocytopenia.

3. Urine with the odor of sweaty feet.

4. **Treatment.** Glycine to detoxify abnormal metabolites.

5. Death usually occurs within the first month of life. Survivors are severely mentally retarded.

## F. Lowe syndrome (oculocerebrorenal syndrome)

1. Disorder of AA transport.

2. X-linked transmission.

3. **Clinical presentation**

   **a.** Cataracts.

   **b.** Glaucoma.

   **c.** Mental retardation.

   **d.** Renal tubular acidosis.

   **e.** Renal rickets.

  **G. Hartnup disease**

   **1.** Defect in renal tubular reabsorption of neutral AA.

   **2.** Intermittent episodes of ataxia and a pellagra-like rash.

   **3.** Fifty percent of patients will be mentally retarded.

   **4. Treatment.** Nicotinic acid.

## II. ORGANIC ACIDURIA

  **A. Proprionic acidemia (ketotic hyperglycemia)**

   **1.** Acidosis, excretion of excessive amounts of organic acids in urine, causing a large anion gap in the urine.

   **2. Presentation.** Vomiting, ketosis, coma, neutropenia, thrombocytopenia.

   **3. Features**

    **a.** Mental retardation.

    **b.** Spasticity.

    **c.** Seizures.

   **4. Treatment.** Extreme protein restriction, ultimately causing protein deficiency.

## III. DISORDERS OF CARBOHYDRATE METABOLISM

  **A. Galactosemia**

   **1.** Absence of galactose-1-phospate uridyl transferase.

   **2. Presentation.** Jaundice in the first week of life.

   **3.** Increased conjugated and unconjugated bilirubin.

   **4.** Galactose is present in the urine.

   **5. Treatment.** No milk or milk products (source of galactose).

   **6.** If treated early, development is normal. If treatment is delayed, hepatic cirrhosis, aminoaciduria, cataracts, and mental retardation occur.

  **B. von Gierke's disease**

   **1.** Deficiency of glucose-6-phosphate, preventing the conversion of glycogen into glucose. There is an accumulation of normal glycogen in the liver and kidneys.

   **2. Presentation.** Sustained hypoglycemia, lactic and pyruvic acidosis, hyperlipemia, seizures, and mental retardation.

   **3. Treatment.** Medium-chain triglycerides and glucose in small, frequent feedings has had moderate success.

  **C. Acid maltase disease**

   **1.** Increased storage of normal glycogen in skeletal muscle.

   **2.** Infantile form presents in the first 6 months of life with marked hypotonia and weakness, including respiratory and feeding difficulties.

   **3. Features.** Cardiomegaly, hepatomegaly, enlarged tongue, and a virtual absence of subcutaneous fat are the hallmarks of this disorder.

   **4.** These children die from cardiac and respiratory problems in the first year of life.

## IV. DISORDERS OF AMMONIA METABOLISM

  **A. General**

   **1.** Disorders caused by enzymatic defects in the urea cycle.

   **2. Treatment.** Nitrogen restriction and supplementation with sodium benzoate, arginine, citrulline, and sodium phenylacetate.

**3.** There is a 92% survival rate, but there is significant morbidity. Patients have a mean IQ of <50.

### B. Ornithine transcarbamylase deficiency

**1.** X-linked recessive.

**2.** Mild symptoms in heterozygous females (migraines).

**3.** Males develop ammonia intoxication with vomiting, coma, seizures, and an early death.

### C. Carbamyl phosphate synthetase deficiency. Severe symptoms of increased ammonia.

### D. Citrullinemia

**1.** Severe hyperammonemia.

**2.** Developmental delay, mental retardation, and death in the first year of life.

### E. Argininosuccinic aciduria

**1.** Presents in neonates with seizures, depressed level of consciousness, respiratory distress, friable hair, and hepatomegaly.

**2.** Older children may be mentally retarded and have episodes of intermittent ataxia.

## V. MUCOPOLYSACCHARIDOSES

### A. Hurler syndrome (MPS IH)

**1.** Absence of **alpha-L-iduronidase** with accumulation of dermatan sulfate and heparan sulfate in the CNS and other organs.

**2.** Autosomal recessive.

**3.** Can be detected prenatally.

**4.** Clinical features seen in the first year.

   **a.** Gargoylism (coarse facial features).

   **b.** Skeletal abnormalities.

   **c.** Corneal clouding.

   **d.** Deafness.

**5. Course.** Death in late childhood due to cardiac disease.

### B. Hunter's syndrome (MPS IIA/MPS IIB)

**1.** Absence of **sulfo iduronate sulfatase.** Excretion of dermatan sulfate and heparan sulfate in urine.

**2.** X-linked recessive transmission.

**3.** Can be detected prenatally.

**4.** Similar to Hurler syndrome in features, but less severe and without corneal clouding.

**5. Type A** is milder than **type B.** Patients with type B usually die before 15 years of age.

**6. Type A** has an increased life expectancy compared with Hurler syndrome. Some will survive into adulthood without mental retardation.

### C. Morquio syndrome (MPS IV)

**1.** Deficiency of **chondroitin-sulfate-*N*-acetyl-hexosamine-sulfate-6-sulfatase.**

**2. Features**

   **a.** Progressive skeletal deformities.

   **b.** Normal intelligence.

   **c.** Aplasia or hypoplasia of the odontoid with atlantoaxial subluxation and compression of the spinal cord and medulla.

    **d.** Corneal clouding starting at age 10.

    **e.** Progressive sensorineural deafness beginning in the second decade.

## VI. NEUROLIPIDOSES

### A. Adrenoleukodystrophy

**1.** This disorder is due to abnormal activity of peroxisomal enzymes resulting in the accumulation of very-long-chain fatty acids in tissues and plasma. There is a progressive demyelination of the CNS, predominantly in the parietal, occipital, and posterior temporal lobes, corpus callosum, fornix, and optic nerves and tracts. Adrenal cortical failure is the second hallmark of the disorder.

**2.** X-linked recessive disorder occurring only in males. The gene is located in the distal end of the long arm of the X chromosome.

**3. Onset** of adrenoleukodystrophy is usually in childhood between the ages of 5 and 10, but may not manifest itself until adulthood.

**4. Features**

    **a. Neurological.** Fluctuations in behavior from a withdrawn demeanor to explosive outbursts, decline in school performance, worsening gait, loss of coordination, vision, and hearing, and seizures.

    **b.** Neurological symptoms precede symptoms of adrenal insufficiency in up to 85% of cases.

    **c.** Melanoderma (increased pigmentation) and vomiting may be the only indications of underlying adrenal insufficiency. Up to 40% of female carriers develop a mild peripheral neuropathy or spastic paraparesis.

**5. Diagnosis**

    **a.** Assay of red blood cells, cultured skin fibroblasts, or plasma for very-long-chain fatty acids is definitive. This technique may be used for prenatal diagnosis and to identify carrier females.

    **b.** Increased CSF protein.

    **c.** CT demonstrates hypodensity adjacent to the trigones of the lateral ventricles with a rim of contrast enhancement. MRI T1-weighted imaging reveals a low signal intensity of the parieto-occipital white matter and T2-weighted imaging, an increased signal intensity in the same regions.

    **d.** Abnormal response to ACTH stimulation is present in 85% of cases.

**6. Treatment** with corticosteroids for adrenal insufficiency is effective. No treatment has been effective for altering the progressive neurological decline associated with this disease.

**7. Outcome** is poor. Progression to a vegetative state is often rapid.

### B. Cerebrotendinous xanthomatosis

**1.** Deficient activity of mitochondrial 26-hydroxylase resulting in a block in bile acid synthesis and the storage of sterols within the nervous system.

**2.** Autosomal recessive.

**3.** Onset of dementia is usually early in childhood.

**4. Features.** Dementia, cataracts, tendinous xanthoma, ataxia, and progressive spasticity.

**5. Diagnosis** is by clinical evaluation and the demonstration of elevated cholesterol in xanthomas or plasma.

**6. Treatment** with chenodeoxycholic acid at the time of diagnosis alleviates some of the neurological sequelae.

**7.** Progression is the rule, and most affected individuals are incapacitated by adulthood.

### C. Wolman's disease

**1.** Deficiency of acid lipase resulting in the accumulation of cholesterol in the CNS and abnormal storage of triglycerides.

**2.** Autosomal recessive transmission.

**3. Features**

**a.** Malabsorption syndrome with failure to gain weight developing several weeks after birth.

**b.** Adrenal insufficiency.

**c.** Intellectual impairment.

**4. Diagnosis**

**a.** Reduced plasma cholesterol and lipoproteins.

**b.** Acanthocytes on blood smear.

**c.** Hepatosplenomegaly.

**d.** Calcification and enlargement of the adrenal glands on radiographic imaging.

**e.** The choroid plexus, Purkinje cells, and leptomeninges may be laden with lipid droplets as seen on radiographic imaging.

**5. Treatment.** There is no treatment available, and death often occurs by 6 months of age.

## VII. NEURONAL CEROID LIPOFUSCINOSES

**A.** A family of disorders characterized by the intralysosomal accumulation of lipid pigments in the CNS, endothelial cells, and pericytes of blood vessels and many visceral organs. These disorders vary by age of onset and rate of progression.

**B.** All are inherited in an autosomal recessive pattern.

### C. Features

**1.** Loss of developmental milestones.

**2.** Seizures.

**3.** Progressive hearing impairment.

### D. Diagnosis

**1.** Family history.

**2. EEG.** Exaggerated response to photic stimulation.

**3.** Biopsy of conjunctiva, muscle, skin, peripheral nerves, lymphocytes, or sweat glands for electron microscopic and histochemical evaluation. Electron microscopy demonstrates curvilinear bodies (granulovacuolar material). In some cases brain biopsy may be indicated for the diagnosis if all other biopsies have been inconclusive and the diagnosis is strongly suspected.

### E. Types

**1. Infantile ceroid lipofuscinosis** (Santavuori disease)

**a.** Early onset at 12 to 18 months of age. Seen primarily in persons of Finnish descent.

   **b. Features.** Progressive visual impairment, myoclonus, microcephaly, mental deterioration, and seizures. Blindness is usually complete by age 3.
   **c.** Rapid progression with survival for several years.
   **2. Late infantile ceroid lipofuscinosis** (Jansky-Bielschowsky disease)
   **a.** Onset is between 2 and 4 years of age.
   **b. Features.** Refractory seizures (myoclonic, akinetic, tonic-clonic), ataxia, dementia, and involuntary movements. Early and progressive optic atrophy and pigmentary degeneration of the macula lead to blindness.
   **c.** Progression to a chronic vegetative state is rapid, but children may survive for several years.
   **3. Juvenile ceroid lipofuscinosis** (Batten-Spielmeyer-Vogt disease)
   **a.** Onset between 4 and 9 years of age with a mean of 6 years.
   **b. Features.** Decreased visual acuity (optic atrophy, macular degeneration, retinal atrophy), dementia, hallucinations, delusions, slurring of speech, and progressive rigidity. After several years, tonic-clonic seizures and myoclonic jerks develop.
   **c.** Death within 10 to 15 years of onset.
   **4. Adult ceroid lipofuscinosis** (Kufs' disease) presents as early as the third decade with ataxia, seizures, myoclonus, and progressive dementia.
 **F.** No treatment is available. Seizures can be managed with anticonvulsants; however, the late infantile variety does not respond well to anticonvulsant therapy.
**VIII. DISORDERS OF LYSOSOMAL STORAGE**
 **A. Niemann-Pick disease**
   **1.** A family of lysosomal storage diseases characterized by an accumulation of sphingomyelin in the reticuloendothelial system.
   **2.** Autosomal recessive inheritance.
   **3. Types**
   **a. Type A (infantile)**
     **(1)** This is the "classic" form of the disease and represents 50% of all cases.
     **(2)** Onset is prenatal to early in infancy.
     **(3) Features.** Failure to thrive, hepatosplenomegaly, developmental delay, progressive spasticity, pulmonary infiltrates, and bony changes.
     **(4)** Death usually occurs by age 2.
   **b. Type B** is manifested by massive visceral enlargement and hematologic abnormalities. Because there are no neurological manifestations seen in type B, it will not be further discussed.
   **c. Type C**
     **(1)** In addition to abnormal sphingomyelin accumulation, type C is accompanied by a defect in the esterification of cholesterol. Sphingomyelinase activity is normal.
     **(2)** Onset is usually between the ages of 2 and 4.
     **(3) Features.** Cerebellar ataxia, dementia, dystonia, seizures (myoclonic, akinetic), hepatosplenomegaly, and

a supranuclear vertical gaze palsy.

   (4) This type is characterized by variable progression.

   **d. Type D** is similar to type C, except for geographic location. Type C is limited to western Nova Scotia.

4. **Diagnosis** can be made by bone marrow aspiration or biopsy of peripheral nerves or lymph nodes.

5. **Treatment** with radiation therapy, methotrexate, and nitrogen mustards have been attempted without success.

## B. Gaucher's disease

1. Deficiency of **ß-glucocerebrosidase.**

2. Three different types.

   **a. Type I.** Adult, non-neuronopathic.

   **b. Type II.** Acute, infantile with delayed development, seizures, spasticity, bulbar signs, hepatosplenomegaly, and increased serum acid phosphatase. Death occurs by 1 year of age.

   **c. Type III.** Subacute neuronopathic juvenile type is rare and geographically restricted to northern Sweden.

3. Presence of Gaucher's cells in bone marrow aspirates. These cells are large and binucleate with a striated appearance to the cytoplasm.

# IX. OTHERS

## A. Lesch-Nyhan syndrome

1. Deficiency of **hypoxanthine-guanine phosphoribosyn-transferase,** causing hyperuricemia.

2. X-linked transmission.

3. Childhood or adolescent presentation with self-mutilating behavior, choreoathetosis, and mental retardation.

4. The increased uric acid causes renal calculi and ultimately death from renal failure. The onset of renal disease can be delayed with allopurinol.

## B. Fabry's disease

1. Deficency of **ceramide-trihexosidase.**

2. X-linked inheritance.

3. **Features**

   **a.** Corneal opacities.

   **b.** Strokes secondary to renal involvement.

   **c.** Intermittent hand and foot pain.

4. Treatment is primarily symptomatic. Renal transplantation alleviates symptoms related to renal failure.

5. Survival into the fourth decade.

# Neurological Aspects of Childhood Disease

Many systemic diseases seen in childhood have neurological complications associated with the disease itself, or as a result of therapy used to manage the disease. The more commonly seen childhood diseases with neurological manifestations and complications are discussed below. Specific management of problems within these diseases is beyond the scope of this text.

## I. NEOPLASTIC DISEASE
### A. Leukemia
1. Leukemia accounts for 40% of malignant disease in the pediatric population. ALL comprises 85% of childhood leukemias with acute nonlymphocytic and chronic myelocytic leukemias making up the remainder.
2. Neurological complications of leukemia are present in up to 5% of children at the time of presentation. In other cases, they develop during the course of the illness.
   a. Meningeal infiltration has been demonstrated in 70–93% of children who have died from leukemia. This may be symptomatic with signs and symptoms of elevated ICP.
   b. In rare cases, ALL may present with neurological abnormalities including seizures, visual disturbances, ataxia, cranial nerve palsies (most commonly VI, VII, and VIII), focal paralysis, spinal cord compression, or increased ICP.
   c. Leukemic infiltrates within the parenchyma may cause focal deficits, seizures, increased ICP, and obstructive hydrocephalus.
   d. Assessment of CNS involvement is made with CT and MRI. LP, if not contraindicated, shows increased cells (often blasts), decreased glucose (60% of cases), and increased protein (50% of cases).
3. Neurological sequelae related to treatment of the disorder.
   a. CNS prophylaxis with craniospinal radiation and intrathecal methotrexate is effective in reducing leukemic involvement of the CNS. Craniospinal irradiation is associated with the development of calcifying microangiopathy, impaired intellectual functioning, and memory impairment. Intrathecal methotrexate has been associated with transient or extended paraparesis or paraplegia, or a chemical arachnoiditis causing nuchal rigidity, back pain, fever, and headache. The combination of these two therapies has resulted in **subacute leukoencephalopathy,** which presents with dementia, ataxia, and spasticity.
   b. Immunosuppressants increase the susceptibility to infectious processes that may affect the CNS (bacterial

            pathogens, CMV, and herpes simplex and zoster).

    **c.** Vincristine (used for inducing remission) is associated with a dose-dependent polyneuropathy.

    **d.** L-Asparaginase (for induction therapy in acute leukemia) may cause intracranial thrombosis and hemorrhagic infarcts.

    **e.** Thrombocytopenia related to bone marrow impairment may cause CNS hemorrhage.

    **f.** Radiation-induced tumors (meningiomas and astrocytomas) are becoming increasingly more common.

  **B. Lymphoma** (Hodgkin's and non-Hodgkin's lymphoma)

    **1.** CNS involvement with Hodgkin's lymphoma is infrequent; however, Burkitt's lymphoma is associated with a 20% incidence of CNS involvement.

    **2.** Neurological sequelae of lymphomas are frequently related to infiltration of the CNS.

    **3.** Increased ICP, cranial neuropathies, and motor weakness are common findings.

    **4.** In some cases non-Hodgkin's lymphoma presents with evidence of spinal cord compression from epidural tumor.

    **5.** The presence of CNS involvement is associated with a very poor prognosis.

## II. ENDOCRINE DISORDERS

  **A. Diabetes**

    **1.** The most common neurological complication of juvenile diabetes is **peripheral neuropathy.** In most cases this is asymptomatic, but can be detected with thorough neurological examination or with nerve conduction studies. When symptomatic, patients complain of pain, weakness, and paresthesias.

    **2. Hyperosmolar nonketotic diabetic coma** is associated with decreased level of consciousness, hemiparesis, and seizures. CNS symptoms are most likely due to a combination of factors including hyperosmolality, anoxia, and altered pH. Cerebral edema develops in some cases and may be fatal. In general, there is a good prognosis for patients who receive rapid medical attention. This condition can be fatal.

    **3. Wolfram syndrome.** A recessively transmitted disorder heralded by juvenile diabetes mellitus, optic atrophy, anosmia, sensorineural hearing loss, ataxia, and peripheral neuropathy.

  **B. Hypothyroidism.** A variety of forms of hypothyroidism occur. Early diagnosis and replacement therapy are important to optimize intellectual and motor development. Excessive replacement has been associated with the development of craniosynostosis.

    **1. Kocher-Debré-Sémélaigne syndrome.** Congenital thyroid deficiency with muscular hypertrophy. Muscle biopsy reveals no abnormalities.

    **2. Neonatal nongoitrous hypothyroidism.** Congenitally absent or small thyroid gland resulting in clinical hypothyroidism. This disorder may not be noted at birth, but becomes more apparent in the second month of life.

Hallmarks of this disorder include an extended gestation, increased birth weight (> 4 kilograms), hypotonia, decreased motor activity, lengthy neonatal jaundice, and enlarged sutures and fontanelles. With development, sensorineural hearing loss, spasticity, ataxia, and poor coordination are common. Intellectual development is impaired.

**3. Pendred's syndrome.** Goitrous hypothyroidism with deafness is transmitted in an autosomal recessive fashion.

## C. Hyperthyroidism

1. Elevated thyroid function is more common in females than in males, and usually has its onset between the ages of 12 and 14, with only 20% of cases presenting before age 10.

2. General signs and symptoms include exophthalmos, goiter, tachycardia, nervousness, irritability, increased appetite, weight loss, and heat intolerance.

3. Seizures, chorea, and hyperreflexia may be apparent.

4. Neuromuscular disorders noted with hyperthyroidism include thyrotoxic myopathy, myasthenia gravis, familial periodic paralysis, and exophthalmic ophthalmoplegia.

5. Improvement without therapy can be seen in up to one third of cases. Medical, surgical, or radiation therapy is associated with a good prognosis. Recurrent symptoms are not uncommon. Treatment results in the resolution or improvement of neurological symptoms in most cases.

6. **Neonatal Graves' disease.** Transient congenital hyperthyroidism may develop in infants of hyperthyroid mothers. This is usually transient, but may require short-term treatment. There is a high mortality rate for this condition in infancy. Survivors may develop craniosynostosis, hyperactivity, and visual or motor deficits.

## III. HEMATOLOGIC DISORDERS

### A. Sickle cell

1. Neurological impairment develops in up to 30% of patients with sickle cell disease. One third develop CNS symptoms prior to the age of 5.

2. Vascular complications related to small-vessel thrombosis and occlusion of the major cerebral vessels are common. Intracranial hemorrhage, subarachnoid hemorrhage, and cerebrovascular accidents occur frequently. Occlusion of the major vessels at the base of the brain may result in reduced capillary flow and the development of collateral vessels (moyamoya disease). As angiography can be harmful, MRI should be considered for the workup of suspected cases.

3. Bacterial meningitis causes 20% of the deaths related to sepsis in patients with sickle cell anemia. Pneumococcus meningitis is most common. The majority of cases are seen in children under 3 years of age. Prophylactic pneumococcal immunization is a useful preventive measure.

4. Fever, infection, hypoxia, dehydration, and surgical procedures may precipitate a sickling crisis and the development of neurological sequelae. Appropriate attention to underlying predisposing factors in the management of neurological problems is important.

**B. Thalassemia**

1. Neurological symptoms in thalassemia are less common than with sickle cell.
2. Pneumococcal meningitis is a frequent complication. As with sickle cell, pneumococcal immunization may prevent this often fatal complication.
3. Muscle wasting, myalgia, and myopathy develop in up to 20% of patients who are homozygous for ß-thalassemia.
4. Spinal cord compression due to extramedullary hematopoiesis in the epidural space has been reported.

**C. Hemophilia A** (classic hemophilia) is a disorder due to Factor VIIIc deficiency. It is inherited in an X-linked recessive manner and is therefore limited to males. Up to 10% of these patients suffer from intracranial hemorrhage with or without associated trauma. AIDS may be acquired through transfusions and result in neurological sequelae (see Chapter 31).

**D. Hemophilia B** (Christmas disease) is due to Factor IX deficiency. Intracranial hemorrhages occur, but are much less common than in hemophilia A. AIDS transmission through transfusions remains a risk.

**E. Polycythemia** causes an increase in blood viscosity, in particular with hematocrits exceeding 65%. Neurological symptoms associated with polycythemia include seizures, headache, vertigo, paresthesias, and visual disturbances. These are likely secondary to a decrease in perfusion from circulatory stasis with secondary anoxia and ischemia.

## IV. CARDIAC DISEASE

**A. Congenital heart disease**

1. **Coarctation of the aorta** is associated with an increased incidence of intracranial aneurysms, comprising up to 25% of childhood aneurysms.
2. **Cyanotic congenital heart disease** (tetralogy of Fallot, transposition of the great vessels, hypoplastic left heart syndrome, pulmonary atresia, tricuspid atresia) may be complicated by the development of brain abscesses, cerebrovascular accidents, and hypoxemic spells (cyanotic attacks). The latter are characterized by cyanosis, a change in the systolic murmur, and a change in the level of consciousness ranging from irritability to syncope. In some cases, generalized convulsions develop.
3. A small percentage (7%) of children with congenital heart disease have associated CNS malformations.

**B. Acquired heart disease**

1. **Rheumatic fever** has become much less frequent with the availability of penicillin. It is triggered by a Group A-ß-hemolytic streptococcal infection of the respiratory tract with the subsequent formation of immune complexes that cross-react with cardiac sarcolemma antigens, inciting a myocardial and valvular inflammatory response. Sydenham's chorea is the primary neurological manifestation of this condition (see Chapter 29). **Rheumatic heart disease** may develop as a consequence of rheumatic fever. With valvular disease, there is a risk of cerebral embolization

with secondary stroke or abscess.

2. **Infective endocarditis.** Bacterial infection of the endocardium usually occurs in the setting of congenital heart anomalies. There is a risk of septic emboli resulting in the formation of cerebral abscesses.

3. **Congestive heart failure** may herald the presence of a significant intracranial vascular anomaly such as a vein of Galen aneurysm or arteriovenous malformation, causing vascular steal and congestive heart failure. Cranial bruits and distended scalp veins are commonly noted.

C. **Cardiac surgery** has become increasingly common for the correction of a variety of congenital and acquired disorders. Neurological complications of cardiac surgery in the pediatric population include cerebrovascular accidents, intracranial hemorrhage, seizures, and spinal cord infarction.

V. **RENAL DISEASE**

A. **Hemolytic-uremic syndrome** is characterized by anemia, thrombocytopenia, and renal failure. Acute renal failure results in electrolyte abnormalities and hypertension that may contribute to the development of seizures and alterations of consciousness. Other neurological manifestations include focal deficits and intracranial hemorrhage due to thrombocytopenia.

B. **Uremia** associated with chronic renal failure is thought to alter cerebral function through unknown mechanisms. Clinically, this can be seen as changes in mental status, asterixis, tremors, and seizures. Other neurological symptoms of uremia are peripheral neuropathy, myoclonus, choreoathetosis, and cranial nerve palsies.

C. **Dialysis**-related neurological complications are not uncommon. **Dysequilibrium syndrome** usually develops shortly after the initiation of hemodialysis and is a combination of headaches, change in consciousness, and seizures. These symptoms are thought to be related to alterations in blood urea that affect the osmotic gradient at the blood-brain barrier.

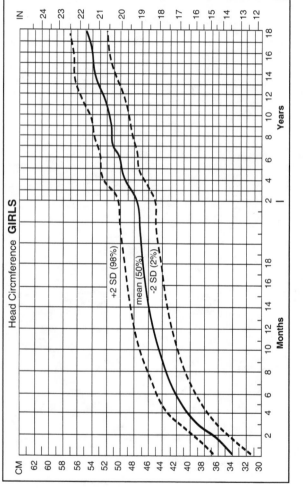

Fig. A-1. Head circumference charts for girls (A) and boys (B). Reproduced by permission of Nellhaus, G. Head circumference from birth to 18 years. *Pediatrics* 41:106, 1968. Reproduced by permission of *Pediatrics*.

A

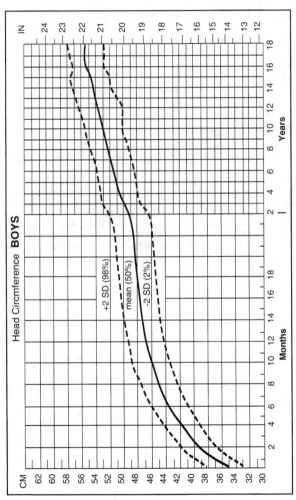

Head Circmference **BOYS**

B

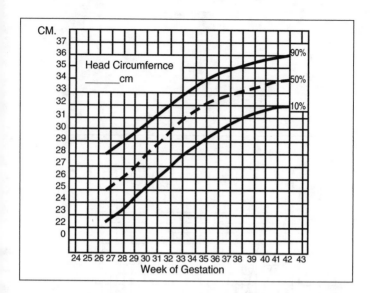

Fig. A-2. Newborn maturity rating and classification. Reproduced by permission of Lubchenco, L. O., Hansman, C., and Boyd, E. Intrauterine growth in length and head circumference as estimated from live births at gestational ages from 26 to 42 weeks. *Pediatrics* 37:403, 1966. Reproduced by permission of *Pediatrics*; and adapted from Battaglia, F. C., and Lubchenco, L. O., *J. Pediatr.* 71:159, 1967. Scoring system reproduced by permission of Ballard, J. L., et al. A simplified assessment of gestational age. *Pediatr. Res.* 11:374, 1977.